the NEW YOU (*and improved!*) DIET

the NEW YOU *(and improved!)* DIET

8 Rules to Lose Weight and Change Your Life Forever

KERI GLASSMAN, MS, RD, CDN
WITH SARAH MAHONEY

RODALE.

To Roo and Bean, Always . . .

Contents

Introduction

'm no stranger to writing about nutrition and weight loss, but when I sat down to write this book, I wanted to do something very different. This time, I don't talk mostly about food. "Hold on," you're thinking. "This is a diet book. If it's not going to be about weight loss foods, what will it be about?" It's about a *brand-new you—and improved diet*: an 8-week, eight-rule plan that will change your weight, your health, your body, and even your brain.

Of course, you won't get any argument from me that *what* we eat is very important (and in Chapter 1, you'll find an amazing cleanse to get you started, and beginning on page 196 there's a full 8-week meal plan, loaded with real foods that are nutrient dense and antioxidant rich). But that's just one part of a successful weight loss strategy. In fact, if losing weight were as simple as knowing what to eat and what to avoid, no one would have a weight problem. At Nutritious Life, my practice in New York City that helps individuals find that "new you" every day, the eight New You and Improved Diet rules simplify weight loss and help you find your way to your best body weight. Each of these eight rules reinforces the others, helping people get stronger, calmer, healthier, happier, more balanced—and yes, *thinner*.

Sure, food is important, and eating empowered is certainly one of the most important things I teach my clients. But another rule is stressing less—and that's equally critical, because stress derails more diets than anything else I know. This book will teach you how a very simple meditation, one that's been proved to lower stress, will actually remodel your brain, making it more stress resistant in just 8 weeks.

Yep—*it changes your brain*. To me, that's not just a big deal; it's huge! Various religious groups, of course, have known for centuries that meditation feels good. And for years, neuroscientists have been able to see that people who meditate regularly have brains that look and perform differently from the brains of those who don't. But in the latest break-through, from a recent study done at Massachusetts General Hospital's Psychiatric Neuroimaging Research Program, scientists have actually documented how meditation changes our brains and have seen on brain scans that just 8 weeks—only 56 days—of mindfulness meditation improves memory, empathy, and our sense of self, and most important, reduces stress. To someone like me, who makes a conscious effort each day to settle myself down through some form of meditation, however imperfect I am at it, I can see what an incredible weight loss tool it can be, too.

I also promised myself I would make this book practical and positive, as well as powerfully effective, in weight loss.

Here's what you'll learn about in *The New You and Improved Diet*: Eight easy rules, which my clients sometimes call the "Keri Code," are explained chapter by chapter. Each rule is connected to and supports the others. The more you sleep, striving for those 8 hours, the more energy you have to work out, the more weight you lose. The more you choose nutrient-dense food, the more motivated you are to exercise, the deeper you sleep. The more sex you have, the better you feel about your body, the easier it is to enjoy healthy meals. The closer you get to eight glasses of fluid a day, the better you look, the happier you feel. See what I mean? I'll show you how to make connections between these eight rules and to totally reset your body's compass.

The New You and Improved Diet provides a simple path and empowers you to breathe deeply as you find your way to the common-sense wisdom that your body already has. Using the healing power of real foods (with an emphasis on fresh, organic produce, teeming with antioxidants), I will walk you along that path, step by step, to the body you were meant to have. When it comes to eating, everyone's "true north" is a little different—this plan will help you find and reclaim your own.

The New You and Improved Diet encompasses everything I've

learned—not just from my studies as a registered dietitian but also in treating thousands of clients at Nutritious Life. This book explains how each of these eight rules is really what your body was meant to do all along, before we distorted everything—before we messed up our palates with lousy food choices, threw off our metabolism with misguided diets, zapped our confidence with emotional overeating, and made ourselves nuts about what we thought our bodies *should* look like. Everyone who comes through my doors, I've learned, is fully capable of finding their own true north, the way they were meant to eat, *and* their ideal body weight. If you simply follow these eight rules, the new you will emerge in 8 weeks.

What does eight have to do with weight? I may not be a math geek, a numerologist, or a big believer in mysticism, but eight is . . . great! The Pythagoreans considered it a symbol of balance. And the Chinese think it is such a lucky number that they kicked off the Beijing Olympics at 8 seconds and 8 minutes past 8 p.m. on 8/8/08! But putting all that aside, I believe the reason these eight pillars have worked so well in my practice is that the number—at the risk of sounding like Goldilocks—is just right. Nine or 10 rules is too many—rethinking your entire relationship with food is a complex challenge, and, well, look at all the trouble people have following the Ten Commandments! It's very important for me to try to set you up for success early on, and my eight rules keep it very simple. And after 8 weeks, you won't just have lost up to 20 pounds and soothed your stress, but you'll have hit the reset button on your whole relationship with food.

We'll cover the reasons you need to understand the power each rule can exert on your weight loss journey. Then we'll move into the second half of this book, an 8-week workbook that provides detailed eating plans, as well as simple tips to implement each of these rules in your life in an easy, effective way. Say hello to a whole new you!

PART 1

How the
NEW
YOU
(and improved!)
DIET
RULES
WORK TOGETHER

While I know you're going to love what you'll be eating on the New You and Improved Diet, food alone isn't enough to change your weight. Shedding pounds requires more than a menu change—you need to change behavior in other areas of your life, or else you won't succeed. I understand that sounds negative at first, but really it's the best news you've ever heard about ending your battle with the scale.

The eight New You and Improved Diet rules, which form the core of this plan, are the foundation of my practice at Nutritious Life in New York City. They truly are the pillars of a healthy lifestyle: It's not that if any one pillar is broken they all crumble. In fact, practically no one I know is firing exactly the same on all pistons. Most of us struggle to keep our lives in balance, even if we spend a whole weekend eating poorly, skip a month of workouts, or go through superbusy times at work. The point is that the more attentive we can be to where we are with each of these eight rules, on any given day, the more balanced we'll be.

I've seen it thousands of times: Clients may follow a perfect eating plan for a week or so, but because they ignore their chronic stress or lack of sleep, for example, they can't help but fall off their plan, despite their best efforts and intentions. Their bodies are so desperate for energy that a whole box of crackers with a whipped cream–covered coffee-drink chaser seems like the answer.

But it works the other way, too. Let's say you have a day or two when you are struggling to stay with the plan, but you manage to get in a long walk and a brief meditation, and you clear some clutter out of your office. All of a sudden, eating that salmon and asparagus for dinner seems like something sumptuous and rewarding, not just something you *should* do.

I've seen firsthand how small changes in all eight of these areas will not only support your weight loss, but also power it and pave the way for, well, *a whole new you.* And as you learn to apply each of the rules to your life, you'll be amazed at how effortless weight loss can be, and you'll get a deeper understanding of why you may have failed to drop many pounds (or to keep them off) in the past. You won't feel deprived—you'll feel *blessed.*

And while each New You and Improved rule ultimately impacts all the other rules, some are more directly linked than others. For example, if you're not eating well, exercise is much more difficult. If you haven't been sleeping enough, it's a good bet your sex life is pretty lousy, too. Throughout this book, look for "How It Connects" boxes that explain some of the most important ways the eight rules feed off one another.

And if you find yourself off track with the plan? Just remember that *every* meal is "Monday morning"—an individual opportunity to eat well. So you messed up and had a slice of birthday cake at the office. Or had two extra mojitos. It happens, and all rules—even these!—are sometimes broken. That doesn't mean you have to keep eating like crazy. Every time you pick up a fork, you get another chance. Changing your relationship with food—really resetting your brain—means learning to be patient, even when you've been "bad." In fact, the essence of the New You and Improved Diet plan is that you get to start with a blank slate as many times as you need to!

Eat More, Not Less

One cannot think well, love well, sleep well,
if one has not dined well.

—VIRGINIA WOOLF

I f you're like many of my clients, you often find yourself so pressured for time that you frequently take shortcuts that make you feel lousy—grabbing a slice of pizza for lunch, skipping the gym, or snacking on jellybeans midafternoon just to find the energy to make it through the day. Yet, at the same time, you're surrounded by more information than ever about what you *should* be doing.

And I don't just mean in terms of diet—although by now, everyone has gotten the message that their life should have much more salad and much less junk food. I mean the explosion of information about the

Eat More, Not Less:
HOW IT CONNECTS

"Eat empowered," I always tell my clients. "The right foods make everything else in your life possible." And it's true: Healthful, nutritious, satisfying, and luscious foods (Rule No. 1) won't just help you get back into your best pair of jeans. They'll also calm you down (Rule No. 2), improve your workouts (Rule No. 4), help you sleep better (Rule No. 7), and stoke your sex life (Rule No. 5).

whole world of nutrition—everything from açaí berries to zinc—coming at you from friends, doctors, TV, YouTube, Twitter, and even as texts on your phone.

Why, my clients wonder, when they know so many of the *right* things to do to lose weight, stay healthy, and have all the energy they need, do they wind up doing so many *wrong* things? I know the answer, and to me, it's simple. But that's because I've spent years watching Americans start diets and then fail. Until we start to make healthier, calmer choices in other areas, sustaining the behavioral changes around food to achieve any kind of weight loss is just too difficult.

Remember, losing weight is hard. That's why the latest research predicts that 42 percent of Americans will be obese—not just overweight, but obese—by 2030. *The New You and Improved Diet* explains many of the things that can derail your efforts and teaches you simple ways to rearrange your life in a manner that supports a healthy weight.

Of course, it all starts with the food. When people begin to understand that eating well isn't about *avoiding* bad foods but is instead about *eating* healthy foods—and not just any healthy foods, but the particular ones your body is screaming for right now—something happens. Honestly, it's like switching from regular TV to high-def: Your entire approach to eating comes into a wonderful new focus. And even though eating is a very physical thing, the shift is almost entirely mental. You develop a new attitude about food, and instead of feeling tempted (or even terrorized!) by "bad" foods, the whole moral dilemma slips away. The New You starts to feel powerful, more in control, more in charge.

It's an approach that works for me personally, too. I've learned to give real food, healthy food, truly *nourishing* food a starring role in my life. And I don't mean that I'm a perfect eater or that I don't know what it feels like to be pulled in a dozen different directions—believe me, I've got a job that can be hectic, two small (and wonderful!) children, family, friends, and my own exercise program to keep up with. Sometimes it does feel overwhelming. And yes, I'm as vulnerable as the next woman to the smell of fresh-baked chocolate chip cookies, especially when I'm tired.

But because I've identified some superbasic ways to keep deliciously healthy foods in my life, I feel good. Most days, these foods give me everything I need to stay strong, slim, and energetic. I can swing my kids around at the playground, counsel my clients, and cook a simple meal—and still have energy left to squeeze in a drink with a girlfriend. Because of the food choices I make, I'm able to ride out the extra-stressful times and the everyday ups and downs and to handle all the good things in my life.

I want you to have that, too. You may not know it yet, but you're about to change your relationship with oxygen—that invisible stuff swirling around you right now, even as it's making its way to every cell in your body. Like so many great relationships, it's got a little Jekyll-and-Hyde action. Yes, we need oxygen to live. It's a component of the air we breathe and the water we drink. Without it, we'd be toast.

But oxygen—and a process it causes called oxidative stress—also causes us to age too quickly. It makes us sick, tired, and overweight. Oxidative stress and the damage it causes have been linked to many illnesses, including heart disease—the number-one killer of men and women in America—a variety of cancers, dementia and other cognitive problems, poor eyesight, premature aging, and even arthritis. And anything that slows that process of oxidation—the same thing that causes an apple to turn brown after it's cut and a nail to rust—doesn't just boost our health; it also makes us feel better.

On an almost daily basis, I hear new evidence—from epidemiologists, cardiologists, cancer specialists, and even dentists—about the benefits of consuming a diet rich in antioxidants. And it has been quite a rush for me, as a registered dietitian helping people learn to eat healthier foods, to discover that fending off some of these problems is as simple as picking up a fork! You heard me: It's not just nutritionists like me who know how powerful a plant-based, antioxidant-rich diet can be in keeping you healthy. Now the whole world knows how powerful simple foods, from walnuts to kale to peaches to cloves, can be.

The New You and Improved Diet teaches you to harness the power of foods rich in antioxidants in a way that makes the most sense for you. Yes, I know you want to lose weight, and you will. But you'll also be eating the most nutritious foods available. (Seriously, this plan is the Fort Knox of nutrition!)

Anyone following this plan will lose weight, if they want to. By starting with the Eight-Foods Cleanse (which begins on page 26), you can expect to lose up to 20 pounds in 8 weeks. Heavier people often lose weight faster, while those with less to lose usually do so at a slower rate. (Sorry—I didn't write the rules of metabolism, and I would change them if I could.)

But my hope is that *The New You and Improved Diet* will spark an even more meaningful change than weight loss and will open your eyes to the big picture of nutrition. It's not so much about what you're going to have for dinner or even the best cleanse for you. It's about nutritional matchmaking. I'm going to hook you up with the healthiest foods on the planet, so that most of the time, they're what you *want* on your plate. (I mean it: You'll start saying things like "Black raspberries, where have you been all my life?")

I'm betting that an internal switch will flip on inside you. No matter what your eating history, you will understand the cause and effect of eating well. Your brain—and your waistline—will really get that these fresh and luscious foods are the reason you look and feel so good. They're not just the secret of your newly visible collarbones (yep, they're there!), your glowing skin, and your softening laugh lines. These foods are also why you feel so great, with plenty of energy to get through the day, a new calm, and a greater focus. You'll be less grouchy, and when you fall asleep, your body will be better able to recharge. Even your sex life will get a boost! (Honest, my clients' spouses send me thank-you notes—a lot!)

I don't mean to belittle your weight loss goals. Overweight and obesity are major problems and cause lots of emotional distress. Many people are constantly upset over how their bodies look and their seeming inability to change, and as a dietitian, I know the heartache it causes. So it's fine with me that you picked up this book to lose weight—and I promise, I'll support you every step of the way. But it's my pleasure to tell you that if all you expect from this plan is weight loss, you're selling yourself way too short. Following this plan will dramatically improve your life—even reduce your risk of the diseases crippling so many people today, including heart disease, some cancers, diabetes, and Alzheimer's. You will eat your way toward a lifetime of lasting, feel-good, and looking-great benefits—a new and improved you! And you deserve it!

Eat Real to Lose Weight

We are learning more every day about how eating real food—often straight from the farmers' market—boosts health and weight loss. Plant-based diets are generating some of the biggest headlines, as researchers learn more about the specific functions of phytonutrients. In fact, I'm thrilled to see the kinds of diet books flying out of the bookstore—*The Paleo Diet, The Mediterranean Diet, French Women Don't Get Fat* (and its counterpart, *Japanese Women Don't Get Old or Fat*). There's one common denominator among these plans: *real* food.

That's because so much of the current obesity and overweight crisis is a product of fake food—not only foods with chemicals and additives and preservatives and sweeteners, but also overly complicated recipes that pile unhealthy sugars and carbs and fats on top of each other in a way that nature just never intended. Until the 1800s, most people lived on simple foods, grown near their home and without chemicals. Local and organic was the only choice they had! And they very likely worked on farms or in factories, which meant they got plenty of exercise.

As more people moved into cities, their diets changed, and an increasing number of processed foods came into our lives. Some innovations—like frozen foods—were great and led people to really improve the way they ate, with vegetables available all year instead of seasonally. But some have been disasters, as Americans have become increasingly tolerant of—and even enamored with—purely synthetic foods. Seriously, can most of us identify a single real-food component of the weird concoctions that made America famous in the post–World War II era: Lucky Charms, Cheez Whiz, or Tang? Does *anyone* know what's in Marshmallow Fluff (which I grew up eating on white bread—really. Mom?)?

By 1971, American eating habits had taken an even scarier turn: We fell head over heels in love with fast food and washed down all those burgers with ever-increasing servings of soft drinks. From 1971 to 2004, a period when the obesity rate went from 14.5 to 30.9 percent, the average woman added 355 calories a day to her diet, while the average man added 168, almost all of those in the form of sweetened beverages.

It's no surprise, when you think about it, that we've become a country with an exploding diabetes epidemic and a landscape dotted with restaurants that have elevated basic fast-food fare to even more damaging levels. It's almost comical to picture what a 19th-century farm family would think if they had to watch anyone eat a Bloomin' Onion, a Chunky Loaded Pizza, a Never Ending Pasta Bowl, or a Chocolate Chip Cookie Dough Brownie Blast Sundae.

Cramming more fat and calories into a recipe has become a sort of scary and weird competition. There's even a dessert called cherpumple that's making its way through gourmet circles. I kid you not, it consists of three pies (cherry, pumpkin, and apple, thus the name), each baked inside a cake (white, yellow, and spice) then stacked on top of each other and covered with cream cheese frosting. Foods like that freak me out. Besides the fact that it has 1,800 calories a slice—more than most women should eat in a day—it's proof of a really fractured relationship with real food.

For too many of us, simple, high-quality foods, well prepared, just aren't enough. There's this sense that food has to be ever-more decadent to be fun. Why else would so many restaurants put things like Death by Chocolate on the menu?

I love chocolate—and I've even included it in the New You and Improved Diet because, yes, it's loaded with awesome antioxidant power. But I don't want to eat desserts that kill me! I want to eat foods that make me feel strong enough to jump rope and play Wii with my kids and go skydiving if I feel like it (OK, I don't exactly skydive these days, but you get my point) and still be able to put in a calm, focused, and productive day at the office. I know that's what you want, too. And this diet helps you find high-energy real foods, with flavors that are authentically satisfying and engineered by Mother Nature.

There's a reason I'm harping a bit on food history here. It's because all these over-the-top foods have seriously warped our thinking and squeezed real foods right off the menu. And it's important for you to understand how these extravagant foods, in a very real sense, are addictive. The latest research from Yale University, based on MRI technology, shows that chocolate can light up the same portions of the brain that are activated in drug addicts and trigger similar impulsive behaviors. As manufacturers and restaurants have layered salt and sweeteners over fat and additives, our palates have changed. We've come to crave these foods, and once you've fallen into the black hole of the Brownie Blast Sundae, it will take a little work to remind your mouth, your brain, and your stomach that a fruit plate—with mangos and melon and berries— is the dessert you really want.

Even many foods that seem simple and real—the chicken products we give our kids, for example, or the "healthy" granola bars we snack on in the car—are often so full of chemicals, additives, and preservatives that there isn't anything real about them anymore.

Of course I wish I could eat all organic, 100 percent of the time, and I wish you could, too. But for most of us, these ideal foods aren't always available, affordable, or even easy to find, and convenience counts. I know our ancestors spent most of their waking hours hunting and foraging, but these days, we have *lives,* which means almost daily we have to make food decisions that aren't 100 percent ideal. Honestly, I'm a busy working mom, so I understand that there are plenty of days when we have to choose convenience over food purity. Especially in airports. Haven't we all found ourselves racing across a concourse, grabbing for a mystery sandwich or a cinnamon bun bigger than our head?

The New You and Improved Diet—based on nothing but real foods, full of natural goodness—will chase those fake foods right out of your life. You won't just lose weight and look great. You'll also find yourself in a brand-new relationship with food, making healthy, antioxidant-rich choices that are perfect for you. On any given day, they'll suit both your needs and your tastes. This is a diet that will become more personal with every food choice, as you discover new favorites and how good they make you feel.

During your Eight-Foods Cleanse, you'll start falling in love with these antioxidant-packed, genuine foods and feel more satisfied than you have in weeks. (This is a *cleanse,* not a fast. You'll eat real food, and you'll eat often.) This will be your first lesson on the power of nutrient density—foods that deliver more good stuff per molecule than others.

From there, you'll move into the rest of the 8-week diet plan and become fitter, stronger, and healthier. And while I can't promise you'll never be tempted by those nutritional disasters again—whether they are blackened, deep-fried, smothered, or whatever—it won't happen often. In fact, you'll be the one in the restaurant ordering the simple dish of salmon and fresh seasonal vegetables, not even envious of the people at your table enslaved by mountains of melted cheese and overly fancy sauces. And after six months of making real foods the center-piece of your diet, you'll never look back.

You're probably wondering how I can be so sure. It's because I know that once that switch has been flipped, there is no going back. Unhealthy foods simply lose their appeal. They start to look less yummy and more pathetic. With so many tasty healthy treats out there—foods that actually make you feel like rocking your favorite pair of heels—you won't crave the heavy dietary choices that make you reach for your bedroom slippers.

Antioxidants Slim You Down

The path from the sluggish pace you are keeping now to waking up every morning smiling, loving how you feel, and liking how you look is clear. Trust me, this is one of the most straightforward eating plans you've ever encountered. But I do need to give you a very short science lesson before we go any further. Don't worry, there won't be a quiz! But until you understand the basic principles of oxidation and how antioxidants work, you won't appreciate the mighty powers lurking in your supermarket and why I want you to start enjoying antioxidant-packed foods—like fluffy brown rice cooked with olive oil, honey-drizzled yogurt, perfectly ripe pears, and even rich dark chocolate—every single day.

First, think about cells, the most basic building blocks of our bodies. The cells in our bodies are made up of molecules, and molecules are made up of atoms. When we're young, and right through our teenage years, all those little bits and pieces renew themselves at a fast clip, and cell renewal is brisk. We're at our athletic peak. Our skin is plump and smooth. Even if we stay up all night or push ourselves in a hard workout, we shake off the aftereffects and bounce right back the next day. Remember when you could pull off an all-nighter, spend the next day at the beach, and still go dancing that night?

But as we begin to age—and I mean as early as in our twenties—cell renewal slows, and cells start breaking down faster. When a cell dies, it releases a lonely little oxygen molecule known as a free radical. These tiny, homeless bits of oxygen are what cause so many health problems.

At this point, my clients will usually say, "Wait a minute, Keri. Oxygen is a *good* thing." And yes, while most know that oxygen is a good thing—and that oxygen equals life—it has to be that beautifully balanced O_2 molecule. Increasingly, we're learning that we need antioxidants to prevent the single oxygen molecules (a.k.a. free radicals) from causing more damage than you'd believe. I like to describe these molecules as unpredictable pinballs careening around inside your body, constantly smashing into other cells, or as someone constantly texting you when you're trying to concentrate. The crazy, unpredictable little free radical keeps disrupting the cell, stopping it from doing its regular job of normal functioning. The fatty acids in our cell membranes are especially vulnerable to this constant barrage. So are the basic components of DNA, which govern cell renewal.

What's exciting is how much our understanding of the process has grown. For example, researchers at the University of Texas at San Antonio have been able to identify the precise way these free radicals mess with the mitochondria in our long muscle cells—the reason you probably can't run a mile as fast today as you could in high school.

Antioxidants work by controlling free radicals through a variety of methods. Here are a few examples of how these clever antioxidants can protect you:

- "Quenching" the single oxygen molecules by destroying them
- Helping the homeless oxygen molecules bind with other molecules in a less disruptive manner
- Preventing the breakdown of the molecule in the first place, so the free radical is never created
- Encouraging the body to crank out more of its own arsenal of antioxidants, such as lipoic acid

In a perfect world, these processes would happen on their own, allowing us to age at normal rates. Face it—some degree of decay is normal and healthy. We're *supposed* to age. And even venturing into the most primitive healthy societies, where people eat pure organic diets and live stress free, you'd find oxidative damage as free radicals built up in their bodies. Aging is 100 percent natural and 100 percent inevitable. And c'mon, it would be creepy if 50-year-olds looked like 20-year-olds.

The problem, though, is that few of us live in primitive societies, and we have lots more than simple aging to worry about. We live in cities full of pollution, cigarette smoke, and radiation. We work stressful jobs that alter our bodies' chemistry for the worse, and then we deprive ourselves of the sleep that would heal us—if only we had the time. Some of us take medications to stay healthy, but they, too, can cause cells to break down. As the free radicals build up in our bodies, the health consequences can become serious: These highly reactive molecules take a toll on our appearance, causing skin to wrinkle and sag before it should. And perhaps the sneakiest effect of all is that when we have too many free radicals, we just don't feel well. That makes us less likely to eat right, exercise, and enjoy sex the way we're supposed to—all the things that keep us feeling at the top of our game.

Unfortunately, too many of us are aging and developing diseases faster than nature intended. The best defense, according to not just one or two but at this point *hundreds* of major research efforts? Our diet! Particularly, consuming real foods, chock-full of antioxidants, including vitamins A, C, and E, as well as dozens of other phytonutrients found in common foods. (You'll notice I'm talking about healthy foods here, not supplements. While I'm not down on supplements, it's important for you to know that taking too many may have some definite downsides and health risks.) Also important are protecting ourselves from the sun and other environmental damage and getting adequate amounts of rest, relaxation, and exercise. And stress management is vital. Each of these has been proved to be effective in keeping the damage caused by those marauding free radicals at a healthy, normal level.

The Right Numbers to Live By
(Hint: Not Calories!)

Over the years, people have gotten pretty crazy with numbers and food. If you've counted calories, fat grams, fiber grams, glycemic loads, and Weight Watchers points, you may be rolling your eyes at being introduced to yet another number. Believe me, this one is different.

I've chosen the foods in this plan based on the ORAC—or oxygen radical absorbance capacity—scale, and during the next 8 weeks, you'll consume thousands of ORAC points per day. (No need for you to count 'em—I've calculated the numbers for you.) It's a scale developed by scientists to measure how well the components of a food mop up the free radicals in the bloodstream.

These foods can help you lose weight, improve memory and cognition, prevent cancer, reverse heart disease, lower stress, and protect your joints. They minimize your skin's lines and intensify its glow. What's more, simply by learning to navigate among these very healthy foods—and feeling empowered by doing so—you'll end up at a healthy body weight. You'll be your smartest, most energetic, healthiest, and most beautiful you!

The idea of using food to corral free radicals is so simple that it's revolutionary. When we eat "empty" foods—a handful of crackers and a soda, for example—our body gets energy from the carbohydrates, of course, in the form of calories. But such foods don't bring anything else to the table. Have a different kind of snack—let's say a crisp Red Delicious apple, sliced, with a tablespoon of fresh almond butter and a cup of green tea—and the picture changes dramatically. Of course, you still get energy, just as you would from the crackers. But instead of a rush of empty carbs (which will likely give you a letdown in an hour or so), you're also getting a blast of antioxidants: The apple is brimming with vitamin C and antioxidants known as polyphenols. The almond butter is rich in protein and vitamin E, along with magnesium and selenium, two minerals with antioxidant properties. And the green tea is packed with something called catechins, which may lower cholesterol.

Many of the foods with the highest ORAC scores are fruits and vegetables. In addition to vitamins and minerals, these are also chock-full of phytochemicals, thousands of which are also known antioxidants. One of the things that makes my job exciting is the increasing evidence that the antioxidants we currently think of as all-stars—vitamins A, C, and E; minerals like selenium and iron; phytochemicals like the polyphenols in apples—may eventually turn out to be small potatoes. There are very likely *hundreds of thousands* of phytonutrients out there!

Every so often, one bursts on the scene like a new celebrity. You've read the headlines, so you know what I mean. Anthocyanins in blueberries! Resveratrol in red grapes! Lycopene in tomatoes! And these do provide us with real breakthroughs in our understanding of how foods work to make us healthier. Much of that research happens in a lab, where scientists look at the actual structure of these nutrients and how they interact, or in the field, where data is collected on the health outcomes of people who consume these nutrients. And it's been revolutionary for people like me. Now, when I tell you why I'd rather see you eat a green like spinach, let's say, over iceberg lettuce, or a fig over a banana, there's real science behind it.

But you should take all of this research with a grain of salt—I know I do. In fact, the USDA, which used to post its research on the ORAC points in various foods to guide consumers to the healthiest choices, recently removed its database from the Internet, saying that there is mounting evidence that there is no clear connection between our health and the specific numeric value of antioxidants. And I get that. There is no reason to start a marketing war between, let's say, blueberries and raspberries, or pecans and almonds. At this point, I'm firmly convinced that Mother Nature was pretty evenhanded when she passed out the anti-oxidants. And it's also possible that the biggest breakthroughs in anti-oxidant research haven't happened yet, and that we'll wake up one day soon to the news that the foods we thought were less nutritious are actually superstars in their own right. Here's an example for you: People have been bashing potatoes for years as an empty carb whose skin holds all the nutrition. It turns out that researchers now believe the chlorogenic acid found in potatoes may help lower blood pressure and that some varieties have antioxidant levels as high as . . . spinach. And sorghum bran—something we think of as hog chow, not people food—turns out to have more antioxidants than blueberries or even pomegranates. (That's saying a lot, because at the moment, the pomegranate is sort of the Ryan Gosling of antioxidants!)

It pays to be a little skeptical, because often those touting the latest health breakthroughs aren't scientists but rather companies trying to sell you something. Some have gotten a little carried away with these claims, and I frequently have to warn my clients to be wary about a quack product they found on the Internet. If it sounds too good to be true, it probably is.

I've based the cleanse and the meal plan in this book on foods with the highest levels of antioxidants, but you should know that our current infatuation with superfoods is a little limiting. While I'll give you very specific suggestions and delicious recipes, know that sooner or later, I expect you to kick up your heels in the produce aisle. Who knows? The green or fruit you fall in love with might turn out to be the superfood of tomorrow (my family is currently having a big romance with bok choy and clementines). The healthiest diets in the world—leading to the healthiest people—include a wide variety of plant-based foods, not just a handful. The New You and Improved Diet is your passport to a whole world of food, not some tiny little salad bar. That's what eating empowered is all about!

As these antioxidant-rich foods make their way into your system—and as your body learns it can count on the steady stream of nutrients you're finally giving it—you won't just feel good. You'll also feel focused. *In the zone.*

I know, all this talk about food is making you hungry. And I promise, we'll get to the plan—which includes three meals and two snacks per day—soon. But before we do, I'd like to go over some very basic eating concepts that will maximize your satisfaction, and your success, in the next 8 weeks and beyond.

Start Tracking Your "HQ," or Hunger Quotient

Finding your ideal weight by listening to your stomach (and body) is a skill many people have lost. We often eat out of habit or to soothe our emotions, without really thinking about how hungry we are. So starting right now, I'd like you to assess your HQ, or hunger quotient: On a scale of 1 to 10, how hungry are you? (1 means you couldn't eat a bite, even if I paid you— it's the way some people feel after a Thanksgiving dinner; 10 means you're so hungry that anything—tablecloths, iPhones, pigeons—looks tasty.)

That's because we act impulsively when we're hungry and are more likely to pounce on anything edible, even if it's not a good choice. Anyone who's scarfed down a whole basket of bread or a mountain of chips before the waiter has had a chance to hand over the menus knows what I mean. But even if we're sitting down in front of "safe" food choices, such as a salad or a healthy stew, we're a lot more likely to overeat if our HQ is too high. Remember, my goal is for you to strengthen the way you and your stomach communicate so you never have that overstuffed sensation, even with lettuce.

So, the next time you sit down to eat, I'd like you to take a deep breath and a few sips of water, and then check in with your stomach. This can be tricky, since most of us are much better at listening to our minds— which are saying, "Umm, that sour cream and cheesy taco tastes good,"— than we are at listening to our bellies, which may be saying, "No más, por favor!" One of the things I've learned working with overweight people is that they are so used to eating past the point of fullness that they aren't even aware they're doing it. Overeating is a skill people need to *un*learn if they want to be successful at losing and maintaining weight. For now, I'd like you to eat until you feel you are at about a 4, the point when you say to yourself, "I feel slightly satisfied."

By the way, I *know* this is hard. If you've been struggling with your weight for some time, that too-full sensation feels really familiar, and kind of . . . comfortably uncomfortable. You're used to it. We need to change that, and I hope you won't feel bad about it, because honestly, while we all understand that it's up to each of us to know when to put down our fork and leave the table, it's not all our fault. There are so many pressures that lead us to overeat. For one thing, there's a kind of conspiracy in the restaurant business. Portion sizes are way more than most of us need, but we're conditioned to finish what's in front of us.

Tracking Your HQ

Each day, I'll ask you to record what you eat in a food journal as well as how hungry you are. (You can download sample food journal pages from my Web site at www.nutritiouslife.com.)

I'll Tell You My HQ If You Tell Me Yours!

1. Stuffed (Like you want to unbutton pants at table!)	I'm never eating again!
2. Extremely full	I couldn't eat another bite!
3. Satisfied	Could have skipped those last few bites.
4. Slightly satisfied (just right!)	I feel satisfied with not one bit of fullness.
5. Neutral	I'm not hungry or full.
6. Slightly hungry	I guess I am about ready to eat.
7. Hungry	I'm really ready for another meal.
8. Very hungry	I'm definitely ready for a big meal!
9. Extremely hungry	I can't even check Facebook until I eat something!
10. Famished (ready to pass out.)	Don't talk to me until I eat—because I may eat my shirt!

Sometimes, our inner cheapskate takes over and goes nuts with that "all you can eat" mentality. I have had more than one client who's been completely undone by Olive Garden's Never Ending Pasta Bowl.

Growing up, most of us were taught that wasting food is a careless, thoughtless thing to do. It's the clean-plate-club syndrome: We were praised for finishing our meals, and sometimes scolded for leaving anything behind. I hate waste, too, but it's OK to want to be a healthy weight. And if overeating is a problem for you, I am asking you to challenge the idea that leaving food on your plate is "bad."

So for the next 8 weeks, I want you to try to stay between a 6 ("slightly hungry") and a 4 ("slightly satisfied") all the time. Let your HQ help you control portions and keep your metabolism revved. Listen to your body!

EAT BREAKFAST

Even if you're not a breakfast person, start your day with something for breakfast, even if it's just a snack. This is the only time you'll hear me say it's OK to eat even if you aren't hungry. That's because Mom was right: Breakfast truly is the most important meal. It gives you energy and lays the foundation for the day. If you're a chronic breakfast skipper, the odds are that you're also not eating well later in the day. I know, I know, you think you're not hungry. The problem is, your body *is* hungry even though it might not feel that way—remember, it's been fasting since bedtime. So by the time lunch rolls around, you're likely to load up too quickly on the wrong foods, especially if you're not in touch with your HQ signals. Now, I don't want eating breakfast to feel like torture—you don't have to sit down to a full meal. You can do wonders just by strategic snacking. Try moving your morning snack to breakfast and having breakfast later.

SNACK TWICE A DAY

This may surprise you. After all, a new study recently found the reverse to be true: The Fred Hutchinson Cancer Research Center tracked women trying to lose weight for a 1-year period and discovered that while those who ate a midmorning snack lost 7 percent of their body weight, those who didn't snack lost 11 percent. But researchers think those results may be due to timing—there is a pretty short interval between breakfast and lunch, and the nutritionists speculate that these midmorning snacks may have been a result of mindless eating rather than true hunger. And in fact, the study found that the frequent snackers consumed more fiber and were more likely to eat fruits and vegetables. And in my experience, that's the power of snacking: Because you never get crazy-hungry, you make more empowered choices throughout the day.

Find the Right Balance

By now, you're probably wondering why I haven't told you whether the New You and Improved Diet is high carb, low fat, or high protein. That's because it's none of the above. The latest research shows that the decades we've spent obsessing about the three basic types of nutrients have been kind of a bust: High-protein diets, low-fat foods, and carb-phobia haven't helped most Americans lose weight. (Believe me, my practice has seen a steady parade of Atkins and Sugar Busters dropouts.) It's not that those plans don't help people lose weight—they do. But the weight doesn't stay off, because excluding whole categories of food is very difficult for most people to sustain in the long haul.

The plan is perfectly proportioned to give you the proper ratio of carbs to fats to protein, while paying careful attention to vitamins and minerals, types of fat, varieties of fiber, and of course, calories. And I've included plenty of produce, foods that are by nature lower in calories, higher in fiber and water, and higher in antioxidants. If you follow the basic building blocks of each meal and stick to the portions I've outlined, you will end up with a diet that is almost equal parts carbs, fat, and protein (with carbs having a bit of an edge)—that's based not just on my opinion, but on the consensus among doctors and many public health and nutrition experts.

PROTEIN provides the body with power in many ways. It is the structural component of all cells of the body. Protein can function as an enzyme, a hormone, and a transporter/carrier. It also provides satiety,

Aside from Tasting Good, What Do Carbs, Fats, and Proteins Really Do?

Carbohydrates	Fats	Proteins
Brain: Chief fuel for nerve cells	Fat soluble vitamins	Hormones
Breathe	Protect organs	Enzymes
Run	Essential fatty acids	Growth and maintenance
Digest	Insulation	Antibodies
Energy	Cell membranes	Fluid balance
	Taste/smell	Blood clotting
	Satiety	Structural: skin, tendons, ligaments
	Emergency fuel supply	Energy
	Energy	

meaning that it helps to keep us feeling full. One French study recently found that by eating eggs for breakfast, dieters didn't just feel more full and consume fewer calories at lunch, the hunger hormones circulating in their bloodstream actually proved the egg protein fully satisfied them: Ghrelin, the hormone that signals hunger, was significantly lower. And levels of the hormone that signals to the body that it's full were significantly higher. The protein foods I recommend are mostly lean protein sources, to protect your arteries.

CARBS give energy to all cells of our bodies, particularly our brains. What good are all those brain-boosting antioxidants if you don't have the energy to use them? In this plan, you'll get the majority of your carbs from fruit, yogurt, and veggies. That means you'll be eating more complex carbs and whole grains, which are often lower on the glycemic index. Expect plenty of yummy oatmeal, quinoa, brown rice, and barley!

FAT is our friend! Despite all the efforts to demonize it, our bodies need some fat to function well. Without it, our skin gets dry, our hair gets brittle, we get constipated—and who likes *that*? A fat deficiency can also cause gastrointestinal distress, menstrual abnormalities, fatigue, anemia, headaches, and even memory loss. Fat helps us absorb certain vitamins and minerals (including antioxidants) properly. We also need fat to burn fat! Finally, fat makes food taste palatable and gives us a feeling of satisfaction after eating a meal or snack.

Regardless of whether it is a protein, a carb, or a fat, each food that I've chosen for the plan is nutrient dense, as well. That means it packs more nutrition per calorie than other foods in the same category.

Develop a Passion for Portions

I'm sure you've seen all the news reports saying that portion distortion has reached epic proportions. It wasn't that long ago that 8 ounces of a soft drink was considered one serving. Then it was 12 ounces, then 16. Every time I see someone walking down the street with one of those 64-ounce cups, I shudder. In fact, even though Michael Bloomberg, mayor of my home city of New York, has taken a lot of heat for limiting soft-drink portion sizes to 16 ounces, I applaud it: It's a great first step toward limiting our supersized soda swilling. Examples of proportion distortion are everywhere: bagels as big as bunny rabbits, burgers the size of birthday cakes. It's no wonder we're all so confused about eating.

And it's not just restaurants. Packaged foods have added to the confusion by listing their nutritional information in as deceptive a manner as possible. Who hasn't been faked out by an itty-bitty bag of chips whose label says 100 calories per serving, only to read the fine print and discover that the bag actually contains 2.5 servings?

As you begin the plan, you'll see that I have carefully controlled portions, keeping proportion of nutrients (carbs, fat, and protein) in mind. By the end of the 8 weeks, you should be a pro at understanding what a meal and snack should look like. A few things to remember about portions and how I have chosen the ones I have: When it comes to fat, starches, and milk or milk substitutes, be careful with portions. For protein, begin with the portion I suggest. If this serving is not adequate for you, increase it slightly, starting with approximately 1 ounce. Listen to your body and let your HQ guide you. You'll notice I only give portions of veggies when they are being used in a recipe. Other than that, I don't give portions because I want you to eat up! Just remember to be diligent with the portion of olive oil that you may be sautéing your big bowl of spinach in. To lose and maintain a healthy weight, you'll need to develop your own sense of portion policing. Ultimately, your HQ will guide you. Keep measuring cups and spoons handy to make sure you are not getting heavy-handed.

Enjoy Real Calories

Moving into the plan, you'll notice I use the word "nutrient density" a lot, and sometimes, it confuses people. Simply put, a nutrient dense food is one that provides a high ratio of nutrients (like antioxidants or healthy fat) per calorie, whether it's a relatively high-calorie healthy food, like olive oil or salmon, for example, or a low-calorie choice, like kale. Nutritionally, these foods offer the most bang for your calorie buck, so to speak. And they are the total opposite of foods that are energy dense, or full of "empty calories." (That includes foods like potato chips, soft drinks, and many bread products.)

While experts are still hashing out numerical scores for this density, almost any method of ranking would turn up the foods that form the backbone of the New You Diet: bushel baskets full of colorful fruit and vegetables, whole grains, lean meats, seafood, eggs, beans and nuts, and low-fat and nonfat dairy products.

Now, let's eat!

Eight-Foods Cleanse

The 4-day cleanse is made up of eight foods—artichokes, avocados, eggs, Granny Smith apples, lentils, olive oil, salmon, and spinach. Why eight? To start, this keeps it simple! I don't want you spending *too* much time prepping. These foods are also chosen because as a group they are comprised of healthy fat, protein, fiber, and water volume and are loaded with antioxidants. And, of course, they're delish! Don't forget to drink 8 glasses of water and 2 cups green tea each day. Rule #3 explains why.

BREAKFAST:

> 1 whole egg plus 2 egg whites (scrambled)
> ½ tsp dried oregano

SNACK:

> 1 medium Granny Smith apple
> ½ tsp ground cinnamon

LUNCH:

> Lentil Spinach Salad (spinach, ½ cup cooked lentils,
>   1 hard-boiled egg, and 2 tsp olive oil)

SNACK:

> ½ cup artichoke hearts
> or 1 small steamed artichoke with a squeeze of lemon

DINNER:

> Salmon Spinach Salad (1 cup spinach, 4 oz grilled salmon,
>   and ¼ avocado)

SHOPPING LIST FOR THE EIGHT-FOODS CLEANSE (4 DAYS)

> 8 DHA-fortified whole eggs
>   plus 8 egg whites
> 2 teaspoons dried oregano
> 4 medium Granny Smith
>   apples
> 2 teaspoons ground
>   cinnamon
> Spinach

> 2 cups cooked lentils
> 4 hard-boiled eggs
> 8 teaspoons olive oil
> 2 cups artichoke hearts or
>   4 steamed artichokes
>   with a squeeze of lemon
> 16 ounces salmon, grilled
> 1 avocado

Keri's Eight Favorite
Empowering Foods

Now that you've learned about the power of the foods I've chosen for the Eight-Foods Cleanse, here are eight additional foods that are at the top of my list for both weight loss and building health. They are included in the meal plan that begins on page 196, of course, but feel free to start eating them even before you begin the plan.

BLUEBERRIES When it comes to antioxidant research, blueberries have spent more time under the microscope than most and are known to be super high in antioxidants and effective in boosting memory, cognition, and balance. Best of all, high-quality frozen berries are widely available—there are always a few bags in my freezer. I add frozen berries to hot cereal as well as smoothies.

BLACK BEANS Besides being high in protein—a 1-cup serving of black beans has 15 grams—they're high in folate and have more antioxidants than any other legume. Sometimes called turtle beans or Mexican beans, black beans are easy to find—in BPA-free cans—in almost every supermarket these days. I love 'em tossed in salads.

CHILE PEPPERS Bright red peppers fuel the fire in cayenne pepper and contain an antioxidant called capsaicin. While the substance gets a lot of attention for its medical applications and is even used as a topical pain reliever, it also seems to have some effect on human appetite. Some studies have found that people who eat meals with plenty of cayenne feel less hungry as a result. It also has traces of folate, molybdenum, manganese, potassium, thiamin, and copper. Experiment gradually, though—adding a few to your scrambled eggs is a good place to start. Not everyone can take the heat!

GARLIC Like so many of the other plants I'm recommending, garlic is jam-packed with powerful antioxidants. Among the compounds in garlic is allicin, which has been linked to fending off heart disease, cancer, and even the common cold. Whose immune system doesn't need that kind of support? I like garlic in almost everything. As long as you don't sauté it

Do Calories Matter?
Yes. And no.

Everyday, I can count on at least one client telling me, "A calorie is a calorie is a calorie, right?" And I can also count on someone insisting that protein and fat calories from the salmon they grilled last night are far less "fattening" than those from a box of Good & Plenty.

They're both a little bit right, of course: Calories do matter when it comes to weight loss. But ultimately, all calories are not the same.

First, let's define a calorie. It's a measure of energy, generated from food once inside the body. And in some ways, it's wonderfully simple: Energy in—energy out = weight loss or gain. This is especially true in monitored weight loss studies, where people are consuming the same number of calories, but from different types of diets. Many studies have shown that people lose about the same amount of weight in low fat diets, low carb diets, or just about anything in between. But to me, that's only part of the story. How hungry were they? How grouchy? How were their cravings and emotions? Were they able to have a social life?

And of course, I worry about nutrients. If calories were truly equal, we would all be able to be strong and healthy eating nothing but Twizzlers. But if we just ate spoonfuls of sugar all day, sooner or later, we'd die. Our bodies need nutrients to function. And foods are more than calories; they are complex mixtures of fiber, vitamins, and minerals, providing proteins, fats, and carbohydrates. Studying the chemical composition of an orange or a scallop or cashew is enough to make most people dizzy!

Some foods have a vastly different impact on hunger hormones, as well as insulin, which controls the way we either burn or store fat. Complicating all that is that our bodies are designed to hang on to our fat stores, making it harder for us to put down our forks.

That's why I focus on lean protein, healthy fats, and nonprocessed, unrefined carbohydrates such as vegetables, beans, and fruit, and whole grains such as brown rice and stoneground whole wheat, quinoa, or oats. Eating natural carbohydrates generally means they are "low-glycemic," so you consume fewer calories while still keeping both hunger and hormones in line. The fiber in these foods slows the release of carbs into your bloodstream, causing less insulin to be released, and translates into less fat storage.

The more sugar a food contains, the higher it is on the glycemic index, and the more it is apt to spike your blood sugar and insulin, which makes us feel hungrier and retain fat. Plus, new research shows that eating a low-glycemic diet is better than either low-fat or low-carb diets in stabilizing blood sugar, limiting inflammation, and helping you do your best, both mentally and physically.

in too much oil, which can add too many calories (I use organic chicken broth instead), add it to any recipe you like.

GREEN TEA Even coffee lovers like me have learned to make time for this fat-melting tea. While white, black, oolong, and green teas all come from the same plant and have similar amounts of caffeine, green tea leaves are prepared differently. Green tea leaves aren't fermented before they're dried, and as a result, green tea is richer in antioxidants called catechins, which may trigger weight loss by stimulating the body to burn calories and decrease body fat. Make your own when you can, since bottled teas have less antioxidant power than steeped teas.

RED GRAPEFRUIT This is more than a breakfast food; it's a weight loss jump start! One study found that people who ate half a grapefruit with each meal lost 3.6 pounds, while those who drank a serving of grapefruit juice three times a day lost 3.3 pounds. (Many people in the study lost more than 10 pounds, without making any other dietary changes.) While all grapefruit is great and has vitamin C and fiber, the red and pink varieties contain lycopene and are extra good for your heart. All grapefruit also contains naringenin, an antioxidant that gives the fruit its bitter taste and that can do the same job as two separate drugs currently used to manage type 2 diabetes. For a change, simply remove the peel—like you would with an orange—and slurp through it segment by segment.

SWEET POTATOES Sometimes I get a sweet craving that just won't quit, and a sweet potato is a perfect solution. A medium baked sweet potato contains more than 400 percent of the recommended dietary allowance of vitamin A and more eye-healthy beta-carotene than any other fruit or vegetable. As an afternoon snack, I'll have a baked sweet potato, with its skin, and add just a little olive oil and nutmeg.

YOGURT This is my primary go-to snack, and over the years, I have recommended it to clients all day, every day. Its healthy bacteria keeps digestion efficient, which is a must for anyone trying to shed pounds. And while research extolling the weight-loss virtues of low-fat dairy may have been a little overblown, the latest research, from Harvard University, shows it does help in short-term weight loss. One my favorite afternoon snacks is yogurt with matcha powder.

What Happens When You Don't Eat Empowered

I'm a really upbeat person, so I don't like to toss around downer phrases like "global health crisis" or "nutrition emergency" unless I have to.

But before I introduce you to the wonderful intricacies of your new "best friends"—I'm thinking you'll be inviting cloves, black raspberries, and white tea over for dinner before you know it—I have to make you understand just how severe our dietary problems are. We've been hearing the phrase "obesity epidemic" for so long now that it has lost its impact. But its huge toll continues to frighten me. Part of the problem is that two out of three people are now overweight, so it's become the norm, and it's what we've gotten used to seeing. We hardly even notice when someone is heavy—that even happens to me these days, and I'm specially trained in recognizing and treating overweight.

But our obesity problem involves much more than all that extra weight. It's sparked near-catastrophic health problems on many fronts. Because of the way our diets and lifestyles have changed, chronic diseases, including obesity, diabetes, cardiovascular disease, hypertension and stroke, and some types of cancer, are becoming increasingly significant causes of disability and premature death, reports the World Health Organization. And not just here in the United States but around the world. By 2020, these chronic illnesses—most either preventable or controllable with better food choices—will be responsible for 75 percent of all deaths.

Here's what you need to know about these major-league health risks—if any run in your family, be extra attentive—along with a taste of what health researchers are learning about how eating antioxidants can help reduce those risks.

HEART DISEASE

This is the leading cause of death in the United States and a major cause of disability. About every 25 seconds, an American will have a coronary event, and about one every minute will die from such an event, reports the Centers for Disease Control and Prevention (CDC). Women account for 50 percent of all deaths caused by heart disease.

THE NEW YOU! Based on many research studies, the American Heart Association now recommends a balanced diet that includes a variety of fruits, vegetables, and whole grains. Tea is also promising: An Australian study found that drinking just three cups of tea a day—green or black—may lower the risk of a heart attack by 11 percent. Researchers think the poly-phenols in green tea may lower blood pressure and cholesterol and reduce oxidative stress. Omega-3 fatty acids, like those found in salmon and walnuts, also protect your heart. And researchers at Tufts University have shown that the compounds in garlic reduce the risk of heart disease.

CANCER

The second leading cause of death in the United States, cancer affects 12 million people, and some 1.64 million will be diagnosed this year.

THE NEW YOU! Many things cause cancer, such as genetics, the environment, and smoking. But the evidence is clear that nutrition plays a significant role in decreasing your cancer risk: More produce, less fat, and as few chemicals as possible are the hallmarks of an anticancer eating program, and the core DNA of the plan. You'll get plenty of foods that have been specifically linked to lowering cancer risks, including soy, fish, spinach, cabbage, broccoli, beets, and even pistachios!

(continued)

What Happens When You Don't Eat Empowered—*Continued*

DIABETES

Nearly 24 million people in the United States have diabetes, and another 57 million Americans are at risk. This disease is the seventh leading cause of death in its own right, but it is especially dangerous in that it also contributes to heart disease, stroke, and high blood pressure and is a leading cause of blindness. Recently, the CDC predicted that by 2050—hello, that's more or less in our lifetime!—*one in three* Americans will have diabetes. Sometimes I look at the statistics and think, "This is nuts!" Frankly, I still have a hard time taking in that one in 10 of us have this diet-related disease now. It wasn't that many years ago that it was a relatively unusual condition and just about unheard of in younger people.

THE NEW YOU! Researchers have discovered that eating $1\frac{1}{2}$ servings a day of spinach and other leafy greens reduces the risk of diabetes by 14 percent. They believe the benefits come from the greens' high concentrations of polyphenols and vitamin C, which have antioxidant properties as well as magnesium. Cinnamon also lowers the risk. A diet rich in natural antioxidants helps people who already have diabetes by improving their insulin sensitivity, and it actually enhances the effect of the insulin-sensitizing drug metformin, the most commonly prescribed drug for this serious condition.

OBESITY

Many experts think we'd be better off if we considered obesity, technically defined as anyone with a body mass index (BMI) greater than 30, a disease in its own right. (Want to know your BMI? Check out the calculator on my Web site at nhlbisupport. com/bmi/) After all, they argue, there's a direct link between obesity—which affects roughly 36 percent of American men and women—and diabetes, hypertension, heart disease, sleep apnea, and some types of cancer.

THE NEW YOU! We know that eating plenty of healthy foods, including fruits and vegetables and satisfying lean proteins, is the best way to lose weight—and keep it off.

I could go on and on, and tell you about research connections between dietary antioxidants and serious health problems as varied as joint disease, dementia, infertility, and asthma. And I could even tell you the ways antioxidant powerhouses improve your body's ability to fend off minor annoyances, from hormonal upheavals to sleep disturbances and even the common cold.

Note that I am not trying to oversell these benefits. As I've said, much of this research is still preliminary—scientists still don't know how many antioxidants are out there, exactly how they work, or all the ways they can help us. That's why I get nervous when I hear companies make claims that their products or foods can cure anything. In fact, the US Food and Drug Administration is cracking down on companies that are too zealous in their promises about what pomegranates, green tea, and açaí berries, for example, can do.

The foods I've chosen have much more than just antioxidants. Researchers are finding that the types of fat, the protein selections, and the whole grains I've chosen will take your nutrition to a much higher level, all while melting away extra pounds.

I just want you to understand how exciting this is, and to appreciate that scientists at universities and government labs all over the world are exploring the healing properties of the foods I'm about to lay out for you. These foods don't just feed you; they *nourish* you. You'll be you, but better—a healthier, more energetic person from the inside out.

Rule No. 2

Breathe Your Way Thin

Smile, breathe, and go slowly.

—THICH NHAT HANH

For years, RDs like me would often chat about how damaging stress was to people's health and talk about ways to manage it. At this point, there are mountains of research showing how chronic stress contributes to heart disease, depression, weakened immune function, and even cancer.

But we didn't fully understand just how big an effect stress has on how much you weigh. And until you learn more effective ways to manage the stress in your daily life, your ability to lose weight—and to keep it off—is really limited. "Ouch," I bet you're thinking. "This

Breathe Your Way Thin:
HOW IT CONNECTS

All of us have at least a little stress in our lives. But few are aware of the way excessive stress can wreck our health: An estimated 75 to 90 percent of all doctors' visits are related to stress. It also derails diets. Learning to handle your stress (Rule No. 2) will help you eat healthier (Rule No. 1), sleep more soundly (Rule No. 7), pamper yourself instead of burning out (Rule No. 6), and take better control of your surroundings (Rule No. 8)

woman is harsh. She's not only expecting me to follow the New You and Improved Diet, but she's also saying I have to be peaceful and serene while I do it!"

Nope—I promise. Anyone who knows me will tell you that "peaceful" and "serene" aren't words applied to me very often. But I do actively work on managing stress—every single day—and this has given me much greater control over how calm (or frantic!) I am at any given moment. And from the thousands of clients I have helped lose weight and from all my years of reading nutritional research, I have learned that until you develop stress-management tools that work for you, losing weight won't just be more difficult than it needs to be; it may also be impossible.

Some of the reasons for that are obvious. When we're stressed, we're much more vulnerable. Maybe we eat emotionally. Maybe we get so crazy-busy with work that we don't eat at all, and then it's 3 p.m., and our energy crashes, and we "fix" the problem with a caffeinated soda and a danish. (I have a journalist friend who calls the crazy stuff she eats "deadline doughnuts.") Or maybe because of a stressful change in our life—even a wonderful stress like having a child—we find ourselves so busy that exercise becomes a remote memory instead of a daily routine. And of course, all those things contribute to weight gain and hamper weight loss.

But we now know that the relationship between stress and overweight is much more direct. One of the major new breakthroughs has been a greater understanding of a chemical called cortisol, and experts are quite certain that it plays a profound role in the stress-weight connection.

You've probably heard of it, and even seen late-night TV ads promoting zany supplements that claim to "tame" it. Those ads drive me nuts, because in and of itself, cortisol isn't a bad thing—in fact, we'd be lost without this perfectly healthy, necessary hormone. Our bodies use cortisol to maintain blood pressure and to stimulate the metabolism of both fats and carbohydrates for energy. As a result, it can cause an increase in appetite. Cortisol is secreted by our adrenal glands most heavily in the morning and at its lowest levels around midnight. That's because Mother Nature intended for us to be, more or less, daytime creatures. (Though I have plenty of night-owl clients who violently protest this!)

Stress also triggers the production of cortisol, which makes sense, right? Of course our bodies want to create extra energy when we're stressed out. That's what gives us the power surge to sprint through the airport when we're late for a flight or to put the finishing (and often inspired) touches on an important project. Soon, our stress levels return to normal, and our body metabolizes that extra cortisol the way it should. Like all the other stress hormones, including adrenaline and norepinephrine, cortisol breaks down naturally in our system. We take a few deep breaths, and our heart rate returns to normal.

When we're under chronic stress, though, everything about that simple, healthy process changes. Because we're continuously secreting stress hormones, the body never gets the chance to break them down and cycle through them. In fact, new research from Carnegie Mellon shows that our immune cells actually become resistant to the regulatory effects of cortisol. For the study, 276 adults were assessed for stress in their lives, then exposed to a cold virus. And yes, those who had been under the most stress had immune cells that didn't respond to the cortisol signals and were more likely to get sick. That cortisol also makes us hungrier. And not only does that cause weight gain—which is bad enough, right?—but it also has an even more menacing effect: It dictates *where* we gain weight. The pounds tend to accumulate in our abdomen, rather than our hips, and this belly fat type is closely linked to heart disease and strokes.

Between the demands of work, family, and finances, the average person these days is juggling plenty of "normal" stress. And it's a struggle. According to the most recent data from the American Psychological Association (APA), 44 percent of Americans believe the level of stress in their life is increasing, and only 9 percent think they handle it well.

But here's the funny thing: Even though we admit we don't deal with stress very effectively, we still think we're somehow immune to the damage it causes. The APA says that 90 percent of Americans believe stress contributes to such major illnesses as heart disease, depression, and obesity. But almost a third—31 percent—say that stress has only a "slight or no impact" on their own physical health, and 36 percent say it has little impact on their mental health. Um, that's what I call a major disconnect.

What about those people who don't seem to gain weight when they're stressed and may even lose a few pounds? Typically, they're the type of people who don't have weight problems. (I know, it doesn't seem fair, does it?) A 9-year study from Harvard University, which tracked 1,355 men and women, found that while stress caused those with an already-high body mass index (BMI) to gain weight, it didn't seem to have that affect on people who had a normal BMI.

Now, along with the normal stress that we juggle on a daily basis, we'll inevitably be hit by additional stressors, the ups and downs that all of us face, at least at some point: a sick parent, a bad breakup, a psycho boss, or a lingering back problem. If we don't have a specific plan to manage these upsets, our bodies will create such a continuous flood of stress hormones that we won't have the chance to process them all, leading to what experts now define as chronic stress.

Chronic stress. Take a minute to think about it, because if you're like me and a lot of my type A friends, your eyes probably raced right over those two words, and you probably thought something like, "Yeah, yeah, I get it. Stress is everywhere." You may not describe yourself as stressed. You may think of yourself as busy. And you probably don't think of yourself as chronically anything—you keep telling yourself that things will get calmer and, of course, that you will eat better. After the deadline. After the move. When your child starts kindergarten. When you finally get an assistant and don't have so much extra work. Like little hamsters on a wheel, we fool ourselves into thinking that the constant stress is temporary, until we look back and realize that we've been saying that for years. And by that point, not only has our health deteriorated, even if we can't always see it, but our waistlines have expanded, too. In fact, I believe that juggling all these stresses is the main reason most women start gaining a pound or two per year once they are in their twenties.

While I can't help you eliminate *all* the stress in your life, I can show how to manage it better. And I can push you to take that next important step: using your stress management skills to melt away the pounds.

Believe it or not, New You Rule No. 1—Eat more, not less—is a huge first step. Knowing what foods best nourish us and support healthy weight loss goals removes a huge stressor from any dieter's life. (Seriously, if we could redirect the number of collective brain cells Americans have burned through trying to sort out good carbs from bad carbs, and healthy fats from evil ones, we'd have cured cancer *and* cellulite by now!)

Eight-Count Breath

Learning the most important way to follow New You Rule No. 2 is even easier. You're already doing it: breathing. And mindful breathing is as simple as counting to eight. Just breathe in while counting to eight, hold your breath for a heartbeat or two, and then exhale, slowly, while counting to eight. Now, put the book down and do it again. You feel better already, don't you? This time, make sure both feet are on the floor, rest your hands on your knees, and close your eyes. Breathe in for 1, 2, 3, 4,

5, 6, 7, 8. Now try holding your breath for eight counts. Now breathe out again, slowly counting to eight.

As simple as this very basic mediation is, it's incredibly powerful. And often the only one I have time for! While I have been a big believer in this kind of stress-reduction approach for a long time—and seriously, it has saved me in many of my worst chicken-with-her-head-cut-off moments—a recent study from Massachusetts General Hospital bowled me over and has led me to intensify my own stress-management efforts and to urge all of my clients to do the same.

Researchers found that an 8-week mindfulness meditation program didn't just help participants manage stress. It actually changed their brain so that they became less reactive to stress. There's a wonderful kind of magic in this evidence: Managing stress makes us feel better, get healthier, and lose weight more effectively, *and* it actually makes us a little bit more stress-proof. In addition to changing the brain regions associated with stress, it also altered brain tissue in regions associated with memory, sense of self, and empathy. What's not to love in that scenario?

By the way, what makes this particular research so exciting to science geeks like me—and part of the reason the experiment generated so much media attention—is that it offered such strong visual proof. The researchers took brain scans of the subjects 2 weeks before the 8-week meditation program began, and then again 2 weeks after it concluded. While the participants spent, on average, just 27 minutes a day meditating, their brain scans revealed significant changes. The density of gray matter increased in the hippocampus, the area of the brain involved in learning and memory, as well as in structures associated with self-awareness, compassion, and introspection. And gray matter density decreased in the amygdala, which is known to play an important role in anxiety and stress.

One of the ripples of the evidence supporting the helpful transformation that comes from regular meditation, even in small doses, is that the US Army has even included basic mindfulness meditations in its required resiliency training. It turns out that teaching soldiers to control their breath, even amid the most stressful combat scenarios, has proved to be enormously effective and helps them dial down the damaging effects of stress.

Why count to eight, you might be asking? Why not 10? Or six? It's a good question. In the thousands and thousands of years that human beings have been practicing meditation, they have had countless methods to choose from. If you decide to start experimenting, you could quite literally devote your life to dabbling in the rich traditions of established religions or any of the newer practices that have sprung up.

And if you've had a meditation system that's worked for you in the past, I heartily encourage you to reacquaint yourself with it! But if meditation is somewhat new to you, start with the eight-count approach. I think it's a terrific place for beginners, which is probably why so many different schools of yoga use it, as do many types of Buddhist meditation. And I'll be honest, there's another reason I think it works so well for beginners. Remember how your mother always told you to take a breath and count to 10 before blurting out an angry remark? At some moments— like when one of my kids is having a meltdown or I'm stuck in traffic—10 is just too big a number for me! Eight is as high as I can go!

For now, all I want you to do is take 8 minutes every day to practice this breathing. You can use an egg timer or your cell phone or just sit near a clock. Sit any way that is comfortable for you—for many beginners, an easy cross-legged position, maybe sitting on a cushion on the floor, works well. If you're more comfortable on a chair or a couch, that's fine, too; just keep both feet on the floor. (You can feel free to lie down and practice, although that is a tough one for me—I'm likely to nod off, and while a catnap is great, it's not the kind of stress relief we're looking for right here.)

Then simply start breathing and counting. Inhale for a slow count of eight, hold a bit, and then exhale for a count of eight. As you relax into it, you may find it easier to hold your breath for eight counts as well, but tiptoe into that part—if holding your breath makes you feel at all panicky or tense, skip it for now. Try to settle your mind and pay attention to what happens. If you're like most people, you'll lose track of your counting as thoughts barge in and demand your attention. (In my own

"Keri, help! Breathing is boring!"

Lots of people, me included sometimes, really fight even this little bit of calm at first. Occasionally—despite the fact that I've read all this research and know better and that I've experienced the relaxation and strength that comes from practicing—my mind will *still* say, like a bratty little kid, "Ucck. This is pointless. I don't *wanna* sit still." But stick with it! Remember, I'm asking you to do this for just 8 minutes a day, not 8 hours.

Be patient with yourself, especially when your mind wanders. (The most serene gurus on the planet have this problem sometimes, and there's even a funny name for it: monkey mind!)

When you notice thoughts or resistance creeping in, just return to counting your breaths, and when you lose track, start over.

brain, they usually sound like "You forgot to pick up the dry cleaning!" or "Keri, you don't have time for this—you should be rushing around finishing something" or "I'm hungry!") Just notice them. It's not that they're good or bad thoughts; they're just passing through.

When the 8 minutes are up, stop. Shooting for 8 minutes a day is an amazing first step. One reason people get scared off by meditation is that they have this idea that they'll need to spend hours sitting cross-legged to get the benefits, and that is just not true: Remember, the brain remodeling achieved in the Massachusetts General study took just 27 minutes a day (and honestly, lots of us spend twice that amount of time scrolling on Facebook). Experts say health benefits kick in with as little as 5 minutes of practice.

Will it make it easier for you to lose weight, and keep it off? It certainly will! And it will do that while also *helping you fight off aging.* A recent study at the University of California at San Francisco enrolled 47 overweight and obese women in a mindfulness-based intervention for stress eating. The researchers measured the standard markers of weight, cortisol, fasting glucose and insulin, and insulin resistance, and they also paid close attention to telomerase activity in blood cells. (Telomeres are the teeny-tiny ends of chromosomes, which experts like to compare to the plastic bits that protect the end of shoelaces. Healthy telomeres help cells divide easily; as we age, they get shorter and more ragged, and experts believe this is one reason age is associated with so many health problems.)

The researchers say they found a striking pattern of connections: The mindfulness program improved the women's weight, stress, eating behavior, and metabolic health, *and* it sparked an increase in telomere activity.

Don't you feel like you just won the lottery? Meditation can calm you down, slim you down, improve your health, *and* keep you young!

Pay Close Attention to Your HQ

As much as I love the way this kind of breath-counting makes me feel, there are plenty of days when I find myself starting to fly into overdrive almost as soon as I've finished. And really, I'm fine with that. It's all about making progress—I'm not auditioning for the Dalai Lama's job!

That's why it's important to remind you to focus on your HQ, your hunger quotient, which we talked about in Rule No. 1. When we're stressed, with all that cortisol racing around in our body, we think we're hungry even when we're not. So at least five times a day—before each and every meal, and the two snacks I want you to have—take a breath. (In fact, it's another great opportunity to practice the Eight-Count Breath. Really, no matter how busy you are, you have time for that!) Now assess your hunger: Are you at a 6 or 7, a sort of "Yep, it's time to eat now"? Are you at a nearly out-of-control 10? Or are you maybe at a 4, still quite content from your last meal?

Working with clients, I've found that making this connection—a concrete HQ number with a stress-triggered urge to eat—really helps people understand how much stress drives their eating.

While you're at it, take just a half second to think about your mood. I admit that the phrase "emotional eater" is a turnoff and makes most of us picture some stress-mess crying into a pint of ice cream eaten straight from the freezer. (I've had a few clients confess that the only time they use their oven mitts is to hold those Ben & Jerry's pints!) But the truth is that we are *all* emotional eaters, at least to some degree. Our moods definitely affect the way we eat, and honestly, I think emotional eating derails more diets than anything else. (If you don't believe me, just listen to the way you chew when you're irritated with someone—I can tell that something is on my mind if I'm attacking each mouthful like a piranha!)

Yes, some people have a much more serious problem and a long history of eating to comfort themselves when they are lonely or sad. But most of us are guilty, at least on occasion, of eating out of boredom—that's emotional eating, too.

So all I'm asking is for you to be aware of how you're feeling when you sit down to a meal or snack. Happy? Frustrated? Tired? Nervous? Make a little note in your food journal. And please don't think I'm asking you to do this for busywork—it really matters. If you are honest about it, for example, you may find that you routinely sit down to dinner in a discouraged, tired mood, and that likely causes you to eat more. Eating when you're in that sort of mood is going to not only throw off your weight loss efforts, but also mask your real problem: You're not doing as well on 7 hours of sleep as you'd like to believe!

Or let's say that around 3:30 p.m. most days, you start thinking about what to snack on, and you find yourself out of your desk chair constantly, trying to find just the right snack. Sure, it could be that you're having a post-lunch energy crash and truly need a snack. It also could be that you're bored . . . not just at the moment, but with your job. I hate to break it to you, but there's no candy bar in the world that can cure that—you need an updated résumé.

Finally, give one meal a day a mindfulness makeover. Eating mindfully, like all mindfulness meditations, feels so weird the first time we do it. That's just because we're such efficient multitaskers! But eating too quickly leads to overeating, as does eating in front of a computer screen, an iPad, or even an old-fashioned newspaper.

So each day, I'd like you to make a conscious effort to eat one meal more mindfully, meaning it should take you no less than 20 minutes. It doesn't seem fair, but sometimes it's the people who spend the least amount of time enjoying their food who wind up with the biggest weight problem. Wolfing down our meals is something that's so habitual we aren't even aware of it—and trust me, since I have little kids, I'm aware of how easy it is to slam a meal on the table and have everyone finish in minutes, then scatter to the four corners of the house. But it's worth thinking like a European now and again: One reason French people may be happier with smaller servings is that they take their time when eating. Researchers have found that even at McDonald's, a chain devoted to speedy eating, the average French person spends 22.2 minutes having lunch, versus 14.4 minutes for Americans.

And in Okinawa, where people have the longest, healthiest life expectancy in the world, they practice something called *hara hachi bu*: That means they eat until they are 80 percent full, then wait for 20 minutes to see how they feel. Not surprisingly, they are among the leanest, happiest people around.

That 20-minute window isn't some made-up, arbitrary time frame. It's based on the way two hormones—leptin and ghrelin, both manufactured in our stomachs and pancreas—govern our appetite. Ghrelin tells us when we're hungry, and leptin says, "Whoa, slow down, you've eaten enough now." It takes about 20 minutes to complete that cycle of chemical communications. So unless we eat more slowly, we aren't giving our body the chance it needs to communicate. (Of course, sometimes we just don't listen—but that's another story, and we'll get to that. For now, let's give our poor stomach a chance to speak!)

In a perfect world, we'd eat all our meals at that civilized pace, instead of bolting down foods we barely chew while standing over the sink. (I know, some mornings I do that, too!) And really, the New You and Improved Diet includes plenty of "slow" foods you can really savor. So sit down, put your food on a pretty plate, take a deep breath—and *mangia*!

Keri's Eight Favorite
Stress-Fighting Foods

Defining stress-fighting foods can be tricky. More than one client has tried to convince me that ice cream is a stress buster! And many people would argue that their personal comfort foods fall into this category. But here are my eight all-stars for stress management: They contain powerful nutrients, such as complex carbs, that help you better manage stress, and they also offer nutritional support to help your body bounce back from the biological effects of stress.

CASHEWS Like all nuts, cashews are a perfect snack, offering healthy fats, calming protein, and enough of a crunch to cure cravings. But cashews pack more of a zinc punch than other nuts, and a one-ounce serving has 11 percent of your Recommended Dietary Allowance, or RDA. And cashew butter is a nice change from peanuts!

CELERY I think this food deserves its stress-busting reputation just for the satisfying way it crunches when you eat it a stalk at a time. An ages-old Chinese remedy for high blood pressure, celery has been shown by modern research to have a chemical (3-n-butylphthalide, if you're curious) that lowers the concentration of stress hormones in the blood, causing constricted blood vessels to relax. It's also a good source of magnesium, which is vital in controlling blood pressure.

CHOCOLATE Besides having healthy antioxidants, this treat is also a mood booster. A recent study from the University of California, San Diego, School of Medicine reports that both women and men eat more chocolate as depressive symptoms increase. While all chocolate has some healthy antioxidant power, dark chocolate in particular is known to lower blood pressure, adding to a feeling of calm. It contains more polyphenols and flavanols, two important types of antioxidants, than some fruit juices. Just keep portions small—I like those one-ounce squares—to keep your weight loss on track.

FLAXSEED The best reason ever to head to your local health food store, these powerful little seeds have a nice, nutty flavor. While the whole seed is harder to digest, in its ground-up form, flax provides a dynamite dietary source of lignans, plant estrogens that may soothe the monthly mood swings that can lead to emotional overeating for many women. And a study from Iowa State found that men who sprinkle flax on their food daily lowered their cholesterol by 10 percent (women didn't get the same benefit).

GRASS-FED BEEF While this costs more than conventional beef, your stress levels will thank you for the splurge. For one thing, it's better for the environment. And for another, it's just more nutritious, with more vitamin E, beta-carotene, vitamin C, and linoleic acid. And while it's lower in fat overall, it's much higher—about two to four times—in omega-3s. One study found that healthy volunteers who ate grass-fed meat increased their blood levels of omega-3 fatty acids and decreased their level of pro-inflammatory omega-6 fatty acids. These changes are linked with a lower risk of a host of disorders, including cancer, cardiovascular disease, depression, and inflammatory disease.

OATMEAL A complex carbohydrate, oatmeal causes your brain to produce serotonin, a feel-good chemical that helps soothe stress. And oatmeal has beta-glucan, a type of soluble fiber that makes you feel full. I love it for breakfast, but it's fine for any meal or snack. I like the steel-cut Irish variety, which takes

"Keri, should I eat before or after I meditate?"

I came across an amazing bit of research recently: Italian researchers fed a group of people a huge breakfast— 900 calories! Then some did breathing exercises, similar to the 8-Count Breath, for 40 minutes, beginning 10 minutes after eating, and some read magazines. Not only did those in the deep-breathing group have lower heart rates, but they also, according to blood samples taken 1 and then 2 hours after the meal, were processing the glycemic load of the meal more efficiently and had less damage from free radicals. Yep, deep breathing = antioxidant protection!

So yes, I'd say meditate after you've eaten. Your growling tummy won't distract you, and you'll digest your food in a healthier way.

about 30 minutes, so I make double batches and just reheat it in the microwave.

ORANGES These are powerhouses of vitamin C, an antioxidant that has been shown to help people recover more quickly from stress. I like to throw them in my work bag or put a bowl of them out in the office. They make the room smell so sweet, and I'm always impressed by the number of clients who will pause, smile, and say, "Hey, can I take an orange?"

RED BELL PEPPERS Juicy, crunchy, and tasty, this is my family's favorite snack vegetable. I like the yellow and orange ones, too, but red

Best time of day to **Breathe Deep:**
Morning

OK, it's a good idea to keep breathing all day long! But on days when I make an extra effort to practice—maybe every time I pour a cup of tea, for example, or whenever I press Send on a big e-mail—life is extra special.

So even though "anytime" is probably the most accurate answer, many meditation teachers suggest that you start by practicing in the morning. That's when your cortisol levels are naturally at their highest, and that makes people feel the most energetic. But mornings are also when you're likely to be most focused, before you get too busy and swept up in the day's activities. So it's an ideal time to start to build and nurture this as a new habit. For me, there's

another incentive: With two little kids, those quiet moments I grab in the kitchen before they wake up are precious—it's the only "me" time I can count on every single day.

Second-best time, experts say, is near bedtime. And there's sound biology behind that: Meditation has been shown to boost the body's production of melatonin, an antioxidant and hormone that helps sleep, by as much as 47 percent.

Some people say that when they start practicing too close to bedtime, they're more likely to fall asleep before they get their 8 minutes of practice in. And while that's not a bad thing, it's better to build the habit when you're more alert.

bell peppers have a higher antioxidant capacity than other types, and higher amounts of stress-sapping vitamin C (providing more than 450 percent of the RDA), vitamin A, vitamin B_6, vitamin E, fiber, and other antioxidants. The unique combination of large amounts of vitamins A, C, and E makes red bell peppers a superfood for many reasons. Your nerves, skin, and immune system will thank you!

What Happens When You Don't Manage Stress

I know I'm not very happy when I let the stress levels in my life get too high. But along with screwing around with our mood, too much stress also has some very specific harmful effects, including:

WEIGHT GAIN

While men and women who are heavy both tend to respond to stress with additional weight gain, women are more vulnerable. Men are most bothered by work and money stress; women tend to pack on pounds if they have strained family relationships or feel somehow trapped by life.

THE NEW YOU! Not only will practicing the Eight-Count Breath help manage your stress, but the nutritious, antioxidant-rich foods you eat on the plan will also help your body recover from stress more quickly.

DEPRESSION AND ANXIETY

Researchers have identified several of the chemicals stress creates that seem to trigger anxiety and depression. Stress also makes the symptoms of both of these more severe. And since depression, anxiety, and related mood disorders are among the major causes of other chronic illnesses, these stress-fueled funks zap your health in many ways. And yes, depression does lead to weight gain and is pretty highly correlated with obesity.

THE NEW YOU! Simple meditation techniques, like the Eight-Count Breath, have proved to be highly effective in treating depression. In one study in the U.K., after just four months of mindfulness training and practicing 30 minutes a day, 75 percent of the participants were well enough to discontinue their anti-depressant medication. (I'm not advocating that, and those medications are real lifesavers. If you take such medications, talk to your doctor about your breathing practice.)

LACK OF FOCUS

Stress often sneaks up on people, and while they may not think they've got a major mood issue going on, they'll describe themselves as flighty, ditzy, or distracted. (I can always tell when it's happening to me because I'll realize I have 11 things open at once on my computer, but I haven't really finished anything.)

THE NEW YOU! One of the most documented aspects of meditation and simple breath work is that it makes people more resilient, more focused, and more productive. (This is now backed by several decades of research at the Center for Mindfulness, part of the University of Massachusetts Medical School, and especially the groundbreaking work of Jon Kabat-Zinn.) For me, the irony is that when I feel this scatterbrained, I'll think, "I don't have time to meditate! I don't have time to breathe!" But the reality is that even 2 minutes of focused breathing gets me back on track and makes me far more functional.

Sip Your Way Slim

Water, water, everywhere,
Nor any drop to drink.

—SAMUEL TAYLOR COLERIDGE

Usually, when clients come to me for weight loss, the first thing they ask is "What do you want me to eat?" They're always a little taken aback when I eventually steer the conversation toward what I'd also like them to *drink*.

Sometimes they'll even ask me, "Is it that important?" You bet it is. We may be oblivious to it most of the time, but the fact is that the

Sip Your Way Slim:
HOW IT CONNECTS

We all know that our body needs fluids to function well. If I had a dollar for every time I've told clients to drink eight glasses of water a day, I'd be able to buy Niagara Falls by now. But hydration is about so much more than hefting that water bottle at the gym or grimly guzzling H_2O at meals. It's about giving your body a steady stream of healthy and restorative beverages throughout the day: teas, juices, soup, and, yes, even my beloved coffee. Proper hydration (Rule No. 3) helps you lose weight (Rule No. 1), makes you look good (Rule No. 6), improves your workouts (Rule No. 4), and reduces your health risk from environmental toxins (Rule No. 8).

water that's constantly sloshing around inside us is very important, not just to weight loss, but also to our health, our mood, and even our looks. In fact, it's kind of funny that the same woman who stresses out because she *only* lost 2.4332 pounds this week seems pretty unconcerned that about 60 percent of her body weight is actually water, and that she might sweat out 2 pounds of fluid in a single Zumba class. Or maybe someone will be up 3 pounds following a night at a sushi restaurant, convinced that the teensy slivers of avocado in her tuna roll are to blame. She can't quite believe me when I explain that even a little soy sauce, packed with sodium, can cause that much water retention.

Many dieters simply dismiss any "water weight" loss or gain as something mysterious and entirely beyond their control, when really, it's as predictable as everything else about maintaining a healthy weight: It is simply basic chemistry and biology.

When babies are born, their bodies are about 75 percent water, and they are already water drinkers. Not only did they just spend the past 9 months bobbing around in amniotic fluid, but they also drank it—about 15 ounces a day! (That's the reason babies have that deliciously plump-looking skin!) But that percentage begins to decline almost immediately, with the biggest decrease occurring in the first 10 years. The bodies of most adults are, on average, 66 percent water, but this number varies according to—and is intrinsically linked to—the way our bodies regulate weight. In obese people, for example, water typically accounts for just 45 percent of weight.

Along with affecting our weight, water is what makes nutrition work: Two-thirds of the water in our bodies is within our cells, where it helps them function properly. And about a third is extracellular fluid, which circulates in our plasma (the spaces between cells) and inside our organs, supplying oxygen and nutrients and whisking away waste.

We can control our fluid levels in several ways, including by how much we drink, how much sodium and sugar we consume, and how much we sweat. But all those things have been shown to be quite variable. For example, the big brains at Gatorade (and believe me, these people study sweat and hydration in ways you and I can only dream of) have found that even among elite athletes, the normal amount of sweat can range from a half liter to 3 liters per hour. Three liters weighs more than 2 pounds.

"Keri, what do people mean when they talk about losing 'water weight?'"

When you restrict the amount of energy you take in, your body needs to get its energy from somewhere, and it turns first to the stores of glycogen kept inside the liver and muscles. So when you use the glycogen, water is also released—roughly 4 grams of water for every gram of glycogen. So, this early weight loss, while important and very real, is mostly water.

After your body burns through this, it needs to burn fat for energy. But fat doesn't have much water in it; it's a pretty dense molecular structure. So while it releases more energy (about twice as much as glycogen), there's little water. That, of course, means slower weight loss but just as genuine.

Drink More to Lose More

While you're following the New You and Improved Diet, I'll ask you to start each morning with a glass of lemon water and then to consume water and other fluids throughout the day, for a minimum of eight 8-ounce servings per day.

Does the number eight here surprise you? As you have no doubt heard by now, the "eight-by-eight" rule we all grew up with has been thoroughly and completely debunked by kidney researchers at Dartmouth Medical School. In fact, it has actually turned out to be a kind of fascinating urban legend. The medical community had been repeating it for so long that no one is even exactly sure where it came from. Many now believe that our national mania with drinking water has gone overboard and that it adds very little to our health. There's even a fair amount of data accumulating about people who overdo it, drinking so much water that they develop a dangerous condition called hyponatremia. This typi-

Happy Hour Advice:
Stick to the Vino and Brews

I'm as big a believer in cocktail hour as anyone, and as you get closer to your goal weight, I think it's a great idea to allow yourself an occasional highball. But in the early stages of this plan, I'm going to tell you to stay away from alcohol altogether. For the first 2 weeks, steer clear and then when you do add alcohol back in, aim to stick to one glass of wine or a vodka or tequila one or two times per week for the remainder of the plan.

Mixed drinks can be especially sneaky. Not all bartenders can be counted on to limit the alcohol to a single shot (home bartenders are especially likely to be heavy-handed when they pour), which may result in you taking in more calories than you expected. The mixers themselves, often high-calorie fruit juices, can also slow your weight loss efforts. For now, it's much easier to practice portion control with a 6-ounce glass of wine or a 1-ounce vodka or tequila on the rocks. And when you reach your goal weight, go ahead and have a mojito with your friends to celebrate!

cally happens when athletes pound water during endurance events like marathons and triathlons. And it's not just dangerous, it's deadly and is now considered to be a leading source of race fatalities.

Most sedentary people who live in a temperate climate can get by with much less than eight glasses of water a day. How much less, though, is highly dependent on each person. Notice two words here that are very important: *sedentary* (someone who doesn't exercise—and as you'll learn in the next chapter, I don't want that to be you) and *temperate*. First, you need to be mindful of drinking enough before, during, and after a workout to not get dehydrated, a problem that is all too common, even among well-conditioned athletes. And second, this is based on people in a temperate climate, which means not too hot, not too cold. So if you are riding a bike in Southern California, snowboarding in Colorado, or even going for a long walk on a hot day, it's not temperate, and you need to adjust your fluid intake accordingly. Even in its mildest forms, dehydration is no fun, causing a dry, sticky mouth, headaches, and tiredness. As it becomes more extreme, nausea and eventually even death can result.

But we're not just talking about general health, and that's not why you're reading this book. Sure, you want to be healthy. But you also want to lose weight, and water can help. Drinking water helps people lose weight faster and keep it off longer. Researchers at Virginia

"Keri, why can't I have diet soda?"

Many of my clients plead, "How can diet soda be bad?"

I believe it *is* bad. Not only is there no evidence that it helps people lose weight, but diet soda drinkers have been shown to be more obese. Second, the chemicals and fake sweeteners really concern me. A recent joint study by Columbia University and the University of Miami Miller School of Medicine found that those who drink diet soda are 61 percent more likely to have vascular problems, including stroke, than those who don't drink it.

And finally: All that fake sweetness messes with our taste buds, so we can't appreciate real food. Shortly after giving up diet sodas, my clients start to appreciate the natural sweetness in foods. And if you miss the bubbles, experiment with seltzer flavored with a little lemon or lime.

"Keri, what about my morning OJ?"

By now, you've figured out how crazy I am for most types of produce, so my clients are sometimes flummoxed when I ask them to steer clear of juice. It's not because I think it isn't a healthy choice—it is. And it's delicious, whether it's ordinary orange juice or something exotic such as fresh pineapple, mango, or papaya juice.

The problem is that fruit juice is high in calories and sugar and deprives you of one of the primary benefits of fruit: all that fiber. In fact, juice is such a big problem that pediatricians have targeted it as a leading culprit in the childhood obesity epidemic and ask parents to carefully limit it.

So while you're on the New You and Improved Diet, avoid fruit juice. Instead, treat yourself to a serving of whole fruit with a glass of water.

Tech found that obese people who drank 2 cups of water before each meal over a 3-month period lost 5 pounds more than those who didn't. And a year later, the water drinkers had kept off more of that weight. Other studies have shown that drinking water actually even gooses our metabolic rate a bit. In one study, the subjects' metabolic rate (the rate at which we burn calories) grew 30 percent for both men and women within 10 minutes after they drank about 17 ounces of water. The gain maxed out after about 30 to 40 minutes.

All studies aside, years of practice have shown me that the common sense of this trumps research: If you have a glass of water when you think you're hungry, very often the urge to snack goes away. It's as though a lifetime of overeating and snacking has messed up our hunger/thirst signals, and one of the very first benefits of the New You and Improved Diet is that your body will regain that wisdom. To me, that is a huge deal, just like learning to savor the taste of real food, minus the heavy-duty salt and sweeteners we're accustomed to.

And while eight turns out to be an arbitrary number, it works, especially now, when you're in what I like to think of as the "training wheels" phase of the Eight Rules philosophy.

Of course, I have met plenty of people who seem to maintain a healthy weight effortlessly and who have made it a point

Best time of day to **Drink Up:**
Before 6 p.m.

For me, the best time to drink is all day, every day, starting with my morning lemon water and ending with a nice mug of herbal tea before bedtime. But since I know not everyone is as enthusiastic about hydration as I am, pay attention to these critical "thirsty" times:

- When you first wake up, even if you don't feel thirsty
- Before sitting down to a meal or having a snack
- Before and after exercising

And feel free to put a cork in your water bottle after 6 p.m. For many people, having to pee too frequently is an annoyance, especially if it wakes you up at night. (Needing to go eight times a day or more, or waking up in the night, may mean you're either drinking too much or drinking too close to bedtime. If it still continues after you begin monitoring it, talk to your doctor. Frequent urination could be a symptom of a bigger medical issue.)

to tell me they don't drink anywhere near that much fluid on a regular basis. And that's fine. I'm glad they know what works for their body.

But be honest, please. If you're reading this book, chances are you're not at your ideal weight, and there's something about your relationship with food and drink that needs help. So, for these 8 weeks, indulge me. Make a point to drink eight glasses of fluid per day, and see it as a step toward both weight management and a healthier you.

And notice, I'm asking you to count glasses of *fluid*, not just water. While I'm a big fan of plain old H_2O, and you'll never see me far from my own water bottle, I do get that not everyone feels the same way. So here's what I'm asking: Start your day with a big glass of lemon water. It will give your body the precious fluid it needs after a long dry night and will help you get a true sense of your appetite before you start your day. (And yes, by all means, have it before you meditate.) The splash of lemon makes it taste fresh and clean and extra refreshing, plus it adds a little squirt of vitamin C, one of the most powerful antioxidants we know.

After that, simply count whatever other liquids you consume, aiming for another 7 glasses of water and 2 cups of green tea. If that seems hard to swallow, know that you can even count your coffee and soup toward that daily 8-ounces, eight-times-a-day total.

Whoa. Coffee counts as fluid? I know, you've probably always been told that since coffee has caffeine, it actually dehydrates you and therefore shouldn't be included in your daily fluid totals. But the Dartmouth researchers—the same ones who officially put the eight-by-eight rule out to pasture—also found that coffee and other caffeinated beverages hydrate you almost as well as water does. So by all means, count them toward your daily total.

Keri's Eight Favorite
Ways to Hydrate

I'm actually a big fan of New York water, right from the tap. But that doesn't mean I don't love other ways to quench my thirst and boost the nutrients in my diet. Here are the eight beverages I love the best.

COFFEE I can't live without it! And that first cup of coffee in the morning, before anyone else is awake, is pure bliss. So I love knowing that it's good for you. Coffee helps wake me up and keeps me alert, and numerous studies have linked it to potential health benefits such as protection against liver and colon cancer, type 2 diabetes, and Parkinson's disease. And it's a primary source of antioxidants for most Americans. But overdoing it isn't a good idea: Although moderate caffeine intake isn't likely to cause harm, too much—more than 500 to 600 milligrams a day—is likely to cause nervousness, restlessness, irritability, stomach upset, rapid heartbeat, and muscle tremors. More important, I worry about it cutting into your 8 hours of sleep. Too many of us (myself included sometimes) use coffee to make up for getting too little sleep. To

SIP YOUR WAY SLIM

achieve the best results on the New You and Improved Diet, just be conscious of what you put into that good black coffee: Low-fat milk is your best choice. Please, avoid all fake creamers and sweeteners.

FLAVORED WATER I know many people find tap water dull, so over the years I've learned a few tricks to spice it up. Lemon, mint leaves, cucumber, and even cayenne all make water more interesting. My latest favorite is adding a few lavender flowers to a pitcher—I love the sweet smell, and sipping it slowly lets me pretend I'm relaxing at a spa. If you're looking for more sparkle, consider investing in one of the devices that lets you make your own bubbly water, and add different flavors. (SodaStream is a brand that gets plenty of good buzz.)

MILK Skim and low-fat milk are a great way to get more fluid and nutrition in your day. Low-fat dairy has also been shown to speed weight loss, and the New You and Improved Diet includes plenty of low-fat dairy options, like yogurt, cottage cheese, and cheeses. If you don't like traditional cow's milk or you have an allergy or an intolerance, there are many great nondairy options I love. I always keep unsweetened almond milk in my home, and rice, hemp, flax, and coconut milks all have their own unique flavors and consistencies, too.

And yes, I do mean skim and low fat—for now. For the best weight loss results, you'll need to stick with the low-fat recommendations I've made throughout the plan. But once you've reached your goal weight, I *do*

Soup's On!

I think of soup as the ultimate comfort food. It can be packed with nutrition—it's amazing how many vegetables can fit in a small bowl! And of course, it keeps you hydrated and makes your house smell great. But slurping soup is also a powerful way to assist your weight loss. Researchers at Penn State have shown that eating high-volume foods like vegetable soup before a meal can help people consume 20 percent fewer calories. Try having a serving about half an hour before dinner on a night when you're feeling extra hungry—I can almost guarantee it will make it easier for you to eat sensibly, and it will boost your hydration! Check out my Web site, www.nutritiouslife.com, for my favorite veggie soup recipe.

recommend working small amounts of whole-milk products into your diet. You've probably heard about a resurgence in recommendations for whole milk, even though it's higher in saturated fat (not to mention calories). New research suggests that after years of getting labeled as bad guys, linked to higher rates of heart disease, the fats in dairy may actually reduce the risk of developing heart disease, as well as colon cancer. And other studies suggest organic whole milk may be even healthier still.

RED WINE It may have been around since woman first crushed grapes, but in the past 15 years or so, wine has become something of a nutritional superstar. Much of the research has focused on resveratrol, the polyphenol found in darker grapes, which is known to promote heart health. And it may also be good for your diet, since researchers think resveratrol may prevent pre-fat cells (called pre-adipocytes) from increasing and from converting into mature fat cells.

SMOOTHIES I think these creamy treats have become so popular because, even though they're healthy as can be, they still feel like a treat and remind me of milkshakes or ice cream sodas. And of course, they're superconvenient for people looking for a meal-on-the-go. I love to make them myself. Feel free to experiment, using yogurt (or milk), a fat (nut butter or avocado), a serving of fruit, and an "extra" such as vanilla extract or mint.

And by all means, throw in some kefir sometimes. A fermented dairy product, like yogurt, kefir also contains yeast, which gives it a different flavor, and it has a slightly higher probiotic value than yogurt. ("Probiotic" refers to the amount of healthy bacteria, which help digestion, contained in foods.) Kefir is thicker than milk but still smooth enough to be drinkable. And research from Ohio State University has found that for the many people with lactose intolerance, kefir may be a better choice than yogurt. As with any yogurt, check the ingredient list—some brands pour in way too much sugar. My favorite brand is Lifeway.

TEA You've already met green tea in Rule No. 1, where I explained how the compounds in it fuel weight loss. But just because green tea gets all the weight loss glory doesn't mean you should overlook all the other delicious varieties. White, black, oolong, and green teas all come from the same plant and have similar amounts of caffeine, but they have very different flavors. And the varieties of herbal teas to try are practically limitless. I especially like teas with hibiscus (particularly Harney and Sons, Traditional Medicinals, and Dilmah). Researchers at Tufts University have found that people with borderline high blood pressure who drank three cups a day of hibiscus-rich herbal teas lowered their blood pressure by 7 points—almost back to normal. It's proven to reduce anxiety symptoms and to promote sleep.

VEGETABLE JUICES Most people's idea of vegetable juice is limited to tomatoes—and I do like a Bloody Mary at brunch now and then. Tomato juice and blends, like low-sodium V8, are supernutritious. A recent study found that drinking 2 glasses a day strengthens bones and can ward off osteoporosis. But thanks to the home-juicing craze, more people are experimenting with all kinds of juice combinations. Parsley, spinach, kale, celery, carrots, beets, fennel, ginger, mint—yum. And, if you are not into home juicing, more and more juice bars are popping up daily. Just make sure to buy yours with ingredients listed above, as these juice bars often sweeten up greens drinks with more fruit than veggies. Also, companies like Blue Print Cleanse that started off doing only home delivery are now starting to show up on the shelves of Whole Foods. Ingredients should be

"Keri, is there such a thing as drinking too much water?"

Actually, yes. Water intoxication, or hyponatremia, can be deadly. And it's most likely to happen to people when they are exercising. It works like this: Healthy kidneys can excrete between 800 to 1,000 milliliters, or between 27 and 34 ounces of water, reports *Scientific American.* That means if you drink three glasses or so an hour, your kidneys can keep up just fine. But during extreme stress—like when you're running a marathon, for example—an antidiuretic hormone kicks in and tells your body to conserve water. That forces water into cells that just can't accommodate the fluid, causing brain swelling and, in extreme cases, death. As long as you're careful to drink only when you're thirsty, you'll be OK!

mostly if not all veggies. If there is juice added, make sure it's the last ingredient. Try one midafternoon instead of your usual latte, and see if it doesn't make you perkier!

WHITE WINE While red wine has gotten most of the antioxidant buzz, in part because of the focus on resveratrol, white wine is also loaded with antioxidants. In fact, a few studies even suggest that the antioxidants in white wine may be more effective when it comes to lowering cholesterol and free radical activity. I like white wine because it lends itself to more spritzer recipes than red does. Try the classic: 4 ounces of white wine with 2 ounces of club soda.

Wet and Wonderful Foods

We get plenty of fluids from the foods we eat—in a typical diet, food provides about 20 percent of our fluid intake. In fact, foods with a high water content, lots of fiber, and plenty of nutrition are the secret weapon of the New You and Improved Diet. And it's not just that these foods help you lose weight. Research from the University of Tennessee found that it's the consumption of these high-water content vegetables that make the difference in maintaining weight loss. Plenty of foods fall into this category, and many are integrated in the meal plan. Feel free to put these on your snack list, or feel extra virtuous when you work them into a salad or a stir-fry. I've chosen them because they are made of at least 90 percent water.

Food	Serving	Total Fiber (Grams)	Water Content
Celery	1 cup (chopped)	1.7	95%
Tomato	1 small	1.6	94%
Yellow squash	½ cup (cooked)	1.8	94%
Cauliflower	½ cup (cooked)	1.4	92%
Red cabbage	1 cup	1.5	92%
Spinach	½ cup (cooked)	2.0	92%
Strawberries	½ cup	1.5	92%
Asparagus	6 spears	1.8	91%
Broccoli	1 cup (boiled)	5.1	91%
Kale	½ cup	2.5	90%

What Happens When You Don't Hydrate

Every year, more than 500,000 people wind up in hospitals for some level of dehydration. Older people and little kids are especially vulnerable, and it can be caused by something as common as a mild case of diarrhea. But lots of us—while not dried out enough to need medical care—are still not adequately hydrated. Here's what can go wrong:

YOU LOOK OLDER, AND YOUR SKIN GETS WEIRD

Even very moderate dehydration can cause shriveled and dry skin that lacks elasticity and doesn't "bounce back" when pinched into a fold. Your skin gets dry, tight, and flaky. Remember, skin is a vital organ—it needs food and drink as much as the rest of your body!

THE NEW YOU! By eating and drinking healthy amounts, you'll notice an improvement in your skin, with fine lines becoming less noticeable. (Clients tell me their eyes look much clearer, too, and while I've yet to find a solid scientific reason for it, it's a nice perk!)

YOU'RE LESS REGULAR THAN YOU SHOULD BE

I think we can all agree that constipation is a pain in the you-know-what. And while it's not a problem you're likely to have following this plan—believe me, you will be eating a lot of produce—it is a condition linked to insufficient fluids.

THE NEW YOU! If I may be blunt, you'll feel better fast, since liquids add fluid to the colon and bulk to stools, making bowel movements softer and easier to pass.

YOU FEEL SPACEY AND CAN'T FOCUS

Mild dehydration often just makes you feel like you're tired, perhaps with some dizziness or lightheadedness. You might even feel confused and get muscle cramps. This turns out to be such a big problem that an unbelievable 75 percent of teams in the National Football League actually give players intravenous fluids before big games!

THE NEW YOU! Because you've got adequate fluid levels and terrific nutrition, you'll be at the top of your game, mentally and physically. The plan will leave you strong enough for any workout you choose.

Don't Get Stuck at the Gym

The longest journey begins
with a single step.

—LAO TSU

B y now, you know how important exercise is to your overall health. You've probably read as many news stories about its ability to make your heart healthier, your mood sunnier, and your waist slimmer as I have.

So riddle me this: If you're a refusenik, why? If you're a sporadic exerciser, what stops you from being a consistent one? And if you're disciplined about your workouts, how come they aren't doing a better job of helping you manage your weight?

Don't Get Stuck at the Gym:
HOW IT CONNECTS

Of course, the connection between activity and weight loss is obvious, at least on some level: The amount of energy we use through exercise offsets the amount of energy we consume as food, so naturally, this rule supports losing weight. (But I must tell you, the energy-in, energy-out arithmetic isn't as simple as many would have you believe, which is why most people need to increase activity and cut back on calories more than they expect, in order to slim down.)

And while exercise supports healthy eating (Rule No. 1), it's so much more than a weight loss tool, and the sooner I can sell you on that, the happier and healthier you'll be. I love that the *American College of Sports Medicine* has launched the Exercise Is Medicine initiative, because I know it's true. Boosting activity levels—even with something as low-key as a regular walking program—reduces stress (Rule No. 2), promotes better, sounder sleep (Rule No. 7), and bolsters self-esteem, which is also related to a more satisfying sex life (Rule No. 5).

The answer: Your definition of exercise is way too narrow.

In fact, the New You and Improved Diet's Rule No. 4—Don't get stuck at the gym—comes out of long experience. Until you find an activity you enjoy, exercise is no more fun than flossing your teeth. If your definition of exercise consists of forced marches on the elliptical machine or lifting the same dusty dumbbells in your basement, no wonder it's not working for you!

The latest research shows that it's not simply *exercise* that keeps us healthy, but *activity*. In fact, even very devoted exercisers who lead otherwise sedentary lives face more health risks than nonexercisers who simply move around more. An important recent study from the University of South Carolina found that people who sit for more than 23 hours a week (and I confess there are weeks when I am sitting behind my desk for twice that long!) are 64 percent more likely to die from heart disease than those who sit still for 11 hours a week or less.

So, if you rethink "exercise," you'll not only be more successful on the New You and Improved Diet, but you'll probably live longer, too.

In fact, as we learn more about the complex relationship between exercise and weight loss, it's essential that you broaden your expectations for what exercise can do for you. It's not necessarily a silver bullet for weight loss. You may even remember when writer Gary Taubes' *Why We Get Fat: And What to Do About It,* debunking the automatic assumption that exercising causes weight loss, made such a stir some years ago. But exercise and activity is the key to greater health.

And while activity, whether it's getting up from your desk for a stretch every hour or going for a bike ride with friends, helps with weight loss in any diet, it's especially true for the New You and Improved Diet, which pays such careful attention to antioxidants and oxidation. Ever notice how every time people talk about workouts, they throw around oxygen-rich words? *Cardio. Aerobic conditioning. Anaerobic training.* What these words have in common is that they all condition the machine (that's *you,* my soon-to-be-fitter friend!) to use oxygen more efficiently, circulating the good stuff throughout your body in a way that exerts less wear and tear on your system. In fact, though we've mostly been talking about antioxidants in terms of the foods we consume, exercise itself is an antioxidant! That's part of the reason people who exercise live longer, get sick less frequently, and feel better than those who don't.

Research shows that staying fit protects our muscles from the aging effect of free radicals. It's actually a very cool kind of compensation our bodies have figured out for us: Exercise, which is by definition a way to stress out our muscles, first increases those free radicals. Researchers have even found them building up in the heart, liver, and skeletal muscles. That should be a bad thing, right? But exercise also triggers our bodies to crank out more antioxidant enzymes, which zap those free radicals as they circulate through the bloodstream, producing an overall beneficial antioxidant effect. (This isn't true with extreme forms of exercise, which can actually create more oxidative damage.)

Exercise is so powerful that it isn't just medicine; it's often better medicine than you can buy from a pharmacist. In recent years, it's been amazing to see the way the proof of that is piling up: Exercise has been found to be more effective than antidepressants, and in some cases, better than blood-pressure medication and diabetes drugs.

Reading that, I know, makes those of you who already exercise feel extra proud of yourselves, and those of you who don't exercise feel a little guilty. If you're in the latter camp, I'm asking you to stop. Yes, I know, it seems odd coming from someone like me, so let me repeat: *If you don't exercise, stop feeling bad about it—there's just no point!*

Remember, Rule No. 2—which is all about managing stress—comes before this one for a reason. I'd rather see you mellow out regarding your decision not to exercise than see you turn yourself into a guilty stress-pretzel!

I'm about to give you a very compassionate way to view your non-exercising status, and I'm not going to call you names. (And if you call

Mythbuster:
The "Fat-Burning Zone" Doesn't Exist!

Not long ago, gyms were buzzing with "fat-burning" workouts: lower-intensity exercises that purportedly burned more fat calories than harder workouts. It's not that there's no truth to this concept. The American Council on Exercise (ACE) reports that lower-intensity workouts—brisk walking, for instance—burn up about 60 percent of the calories used from fat, versus 35 percent from higher-intensity activities like running. But since higher-intensity activities burn so many more calories, you're still better off doing a harder workout.

ACE puts it this way: If you perform 30 minutes of low-intensity aerobic exercise, you'll burn approximately 200 calories—about 120 calories (or 60 percent) of which come from stored fat. But if you exercise for the same amount of time at a high intensity, you'll smoke 400 calories—about 140 calories from stored fat.

yourself things like Slacker, Slug, or Couch Potato, please stop!) Name-calling doesn't motivate people. In fact, there's a good chance that even if I told you exercising would give you Bill Gates's money and Gisele Bündchen's body, you'd *still* say, "I don't care, Keri! I just hate to exercise!" That's OK! Really, I have heard every reason under the sun: *I hate to sweat. They don't make sneakers with high heels. I was traumatized by the rope-climb test in middle school. Yoga gives me gas. I hate those grunting noises some people make when they lift weights. It hurts . . .*

Sometimes, clients will even say, "I'll gain weight if I exercise—working out makes me hungry!" Actually, that idea, as logical as it sounds, is still a matter of considerable debate among researchers. A British study, for example, tracked people after running and weight training sessions, and found that several hours after the workout, the participants were still somewhat less hungry than when they hadn't exercised. The exercise sessions even lowered their levels of ghrelin, a hormone associated with hunger. Other studies have found the reverse, especially among obese people who aren't used to much exercise at all. What that tells me is that we each need to pay close attention to our HQ after we exercise, and see if we have to adjust our eating accordingly. I've worked closely with professional athletes, as well as people training for big events such as triathlons and marathons, and you better believe that they have to adjust their diet to support very intense training.

You don't have to exercise to lose weight on the New You and Improved Diet: Exercise is not the silver bullet of a weight loss program. Some of my most gym-o-phobic clients are quick to point that out! Especially if they've had short-term success with a diet in the past, they will often say, "Cutting back on what I eat works way better than situps!" Again, I won't lie to you—there *is* some truth to that. Studies have shown that people who diet but don't exercise are somewhat more likely to succeed at weight loss than people who exercise more but don't modify their diet.

But you don't have to choose between the two! And I believe that once you wrap your brain around Rule No. 4—to stop dreading the gym and

"Keri, how much water do I really need for my workouts?"

As you read in Rule No. 3, there's been a lot of debate about the appropriate level of hydration before, during, and after a workout. Some people are like camels and want to guzzle liters of water all day; others have to be reminded to take a sip. The big secret, despite all the ounce-to-weight formulas you hear kicked around? It really depends on you: your needs, your sport, your intensity level—and the weather.

The American College of Sports Medicine says it's important to drink an adequate level of water several hours before, during, and after exercise. And I like all my clients to drink at least 64 ounces a day. Hydration isn't important just during exercise;

(continued)

start thinking of activities you enjoy, whether they're dancing, shopping, or playing with your dog—you'll find the solution that works best for you.

It's pretty hard to argue against it, especially when you stack up all the evidence: that exercise is a known antioxidant and a powerful weight loss tool and that it helps you live longer, feel better, age more gracefully, avoid all kinds of medications, relax more, sleep more soundly and even have better sex. Still, about 60 percent of American adults either don't work out at all or don't work out enough to be considered regular exercisers.

That statistic shocks public health experts, but it doesn't surprise me or any other dietitian—or personal trainer, for that matter—who works with actual human beings, with busy lives and all kinds of obstacles to fitness. Exercise may very well be the wonder drug, but translating that knowledge into behavior is tricky: Working out is a difficult habit to build and an easy one to break.

So, if you are among the 60 percent who don't work out regularly—before I talk any more about exercise, or sing the praises of yoga, Spinning, and a good old treadmill— I'd like you to take this little quiz. It's based on a body of research that has been building since the mid-1990s, when experts from the University of Rhode Island first published these breakthrough ideas about how people actually go about changing their behavior.

The technical name is the transtheoretical model of behavior change, and while it's a mouthful, it helps us understand why we often don't act the way we say we want to (as in "Why did I eat a burrito bigger than my head when I swore I'd have a salad?" or "I even put on my running shoes! So why did I head straight for the couch instead of the elliptical?"). It's because readiness to make a change doesn't happen overnight—it often takes years. Seriously. Most former smokers, for example, spend a few years working up to the decision to commit to quitting, and then it takes them an average of five attempts to quit before they are able to stop smoking for good. Are they weak? No! They just weren't as ready as they thought they were.

Using this fitness readiness scale will make it much easier to be compassionate. You can accurately gauge whether you're ready to make a change, instead of beating yourself up and name-calling if you don't. Where do you fall?

1. **NO WAY, JOSE.** No matter what, you don't want to exercise, and you have your reasons—it's a big pain in the neck, it makes you sore, you'd rather read a good book, you don't have the time . . . OK, I get it! Very determined anti-exercisers, please skip to Rule No. 5, with my blessing. But I hope you'll

(continued)

water is critical to all the body's systems, including how well you are able to metabolize food.

So if you're already a big water drinker, mazel tov. If not, make a conscious effort to drink at least 12 to 20 ounces a few hours before you exercise. Then during exercise, drink 8 to 10 ounces of fluid for every 15 to 20 minutes of moderate-intensity physical activity. And take a good long drink at the end of your workout. Many people say that the more they drink, the more focused they are during workouts.

And as always, pay attention to how you feel: Headaches, dizziness, and feeling distracted are among the first signs of dehydration.

While sports drinks do replace electrolytes, you don't need these drinks unless you're intensely working out for longer than 60 minutes. Otherwise, good old water works well and has no added calories.

come back to this chapter in 6 months or so, because things change. Moderately determined excuse makers? Please keep reading!

2. **WELL, IT'S CROSSED MY MIND, BUT I'M IN NO RUSH.** This phase is called pre-contemplation, and experts estimate that about 40 percent of nonexercisers fall into this category. You really don't intend to change your behavior, at least for the next 6 months, but you aren't ruling it out entirely, either. You're not ready to join the gym, but you're at least contemplating getting fitter.

3. **OK, I AM WILLING TO CONSIDER IT.** Again, about 40 percent of nonexercisers (or smokers, or those on the verge of just about any big behavioral change) fall in this group. Usually, the people in this group see themselves as ready to make a big change within 6 months.

4. **WHAT DO I NEED TO DO TO GET STARTED?** This preparation stage accounts for the remaining 20 percent of those considering making a lifestyle change. Once you make it this far, you're probably asking friends questions about their workouts, noticing new fitness trends, maybe even checking out new exercise clothes. Most people who've reached this point see themselves actually lacing up their sneakers within a month.

5. **LOOK AT ME—I'M DOING IT!** This action phase means that the new behavior is being built into your routine—albeit not perfectly—for about 6 months.

Mobile You: *Fitness on the Go*

Since I travel fairly often for work, I know how air travel and rescheduled meetings can derail an exercise plan. Here's what helps: Pack a jump rope and a resistance band—they can fit in even the most overstuffed suitcase. Then if your hotel doesn't have a gym, you can still get in a reasonable workout. And travel in comfortable shoes. Airports offer plenty of opportunities for walking, and a few laps around Terminal A can take the place of a gym workout.

6. I DON'T KNOW HOW I FIT IT IN. I JUST DO IT. After 6 months of any new behavior, the likelihood of reverting back to old habits decreases. We stick with the change because we like the change.

I have to admit, I'm one of the lucky ones—I've loved sports and working out my whole life, so this rule is easier for me. And no, I'm not a fitness saint. I blow off situps and rarely spend the time I probably should to stretch after my runs. Days can get so crazy-busy that there just isn't room for any kind of exercise, except a little wrestling with the kids. But because I have been committed to exercise for so long—I played lacrosse in high school and college, and one of my proudest moments was finishing the New York City Marathon—I know I'm in a good workout routine when something gets in the way of exercise, I feel almost as gross as if I didn't brush my teeth.

All this means is that I've built the habit of exercise, and like any other habit, you can, too. It's just a matter of finding the right activity and the right schedule.

And does that commitment connect to maintaining a healthy weight? You bet your kettlebells it does. Members of the National Weight Control Registry, an elite group whose members have maintained an average weight loss of 66 pounds for an average of 5 years, tend to exercise an hour a day, five to six times a week. (And again, understand that people who are committed enough to exercise every day are indeed a truly elite group: Only 5 percent of Americans do so, reports the *American Journal of Preventive Medicine*.)

And no, I'm not expecting you to exercise that much. But if you're working your way along the readiness scale toward regular exercise (to experts, "regular exercise" means four times a week), I'm asking you to trust me. Once you taste the real thrill that comes from exercise—not just noticing that you have biceps or that your jeans suddenly feel looser, but also realizing that you can run up a flight of stairs without getting winded—the motivation to strengthen that habit will get more and more intense. You won't wanna skip a workout, and you'll be like me—loving weekends because you get to spend a little more time in your running capris.

That will speed your success on the New You and Improved Diet in several ways. First, people who work out tend to crave healthier foods, not junk. (Really, after leaving a Spin class, you're more motivated to grab a green juice versus a cupcake.) Second, it takes more fuel to power your muscles than it does to power fat. So the more muscle you build, the more calories you burn—not just during workouts but even while you sleep.

And even if you're already a semi-regular exerciser, rethinking a few things in your routine can radically increase your fitness level, which in turn will make everything else about the plan work better. It can turn you from a metabolic minivan (perfectly respectable, but nothing to brag about) to a Porsche!

So browse through the next few pages with an open mind, and accept that what sounds a little intense now may feel like an easy workout in a month or two. And no matter what level you're at, keep in mind that you can always vary the intensity—going light on days when you need a break or upping the activity level when you feel the power to make the pounds come off faster. Even better? You'll feel ready to conquer the world.

Workout Plan 1

EASING BACK INTO EXERCISE

Let's say you've tried to stick with a workout routine before—maybe more times than you can count. First of all, don't judge yourself because you've dropped out of a few gyms or routines in your life. The fitness industry, which knows that the dropout rate is high, also bears some of the responsibility. "The fitness community often promises beginners things that can't happen," says Debra Mazda, a Philadelphia-based exercise physiologist and creator of Shapely Girl Fitness, who specializes in working with plus-size women.

First, many gyms—not to mention those goofy devices sold on TV—have overpromised what they can deliver. "You just aren't going to get six-pack abs in 5 days," she says. "So people wind up sore and discouraged, making it easy to quit." To make sure that doesn't happen to you . . .

FIND YOUR BENCHMARK. Trainers suggest that you make your first priority documenting where you are now. Ideally, you should see a doctor if you haven't had a checkup in a while. (If you're like me, you're probably a little suspicious that the "Check with your doctor before starting any exercise program" line is just a little legal weaseling to avoid lawsuits, but it's actually because there are people who are at risk. It doesn't hurt to be checked out to make sure you're not one of them.)

ASK YOUR DOCTOR TO CHECK YOUR BLOOD PRESSURE, CHOLESTEROL LEVELS, AND BLOOD SUGAR, AND TO WRITE THEM DOWN FOR YOU. Once you've got these numbers, write your weight and some other key measurements on the same piece of paper: your waist and hips, along with your chest, biceps, thighs, and calves. If you're joining a gym or already belong to one, ask to have your body-fat percentage calculated.

And finally—I know you won't like this one, but do it anyway . . .

"Keri, should I eat before or after I exercise?"

If it works for your schedule, eat afterward. (But many people like to have something light beforehand. A healthy 150-calorie snack, like a banana with a teaspoon of nut butter is ideal.) That's because a good workout primes the body for maximum nutrition: Not only can your muscles better absorb the antioxidant-rich nutrients you're going to give them, but glycogen—the form of carbohydrate stores we burn during exercise—is also replaced more efficiently.

You'll also burn more fat: The latest research shows that morning exercisers who put off breakfast until after a cycling workout burned off a higher ratio of fat to carbohydrates than those who ate breakfast before working out.

GET INTO YOUR GYM CLOTHES AND ASK SOMEONE TO SNAP A FEW PHOTOS OF YOU. You are probably thinking, "This woman is evil, asking for photographic evidence *before* I start exercising!" But work with me here: This is your "before" moment, and the better you can document it, the more you will thank me later. *I* know exercise will change your body, but nothing will hammer that point home to *you* as effectively as realizing that you aren't just losing weight but also building muscle, sculpting a better body, and improving the actual composition of your blood. Seriously, "before" and "after" pictures say way more than a thousand words!

And the change will start fast. For one thing, as Kelli Calabrese, an exercise physiologist and personal trainer in Texas, points out, once people make the decision to start working out, they typically feel a little better as exercise produces endorphins that make them feel good. "And within the first week, most people notice an improvement in energy levels, which continues into the second week when they also begin to lose inches and pounds," she says. "By the fourth week, they're noticeably losing inches and can see improved definition." By the sixth week? "Sedentary people who have been working out three to four times a week will likely have lost up to 6 pounds with exercise alone." If they make healthy changes to their diet, it can be as much as 15 to 20 pounds. Studies have shown that simply adding weight training—again, without cutting a single calorie—can help you lower your overall body fat by 3 percentage points.

More important, Calabrese adds, "It's also likely that you'll have lowered your resting heart rate to 10 beats per minute and lowered your systolic blood pressure by 10 mmttg."

Still not convinced? A recent study showed that sedentary women who took moderate aerobics classes had measurably lower levels of stress hormones in their blood. Your doctor will probably have one word for this change: *Wowza.*

PICK AN ACTIVITY THAT WORKS FOR YOU. There's no reason you have to join a gym, of course. There are plenty of workouts you can do on your own, like walking or using equipment at home, and there are thousands of great workout videos online. Plus, plenty of other places offer workouts—many adult-ed programs, for example, have cheap introductory classes in everything from dancing to weight lifting; these classes are a great way to stick your toe in the workout water without a big financial commitment. You can find great workouts that take you outdoors—hiking, kayaking, or riding a bicycle.

But if you think you do want to join a gym or a yoga or Pilates studio, that's a good thing, too—as long as you pick one you'll actually use! Gyms put plenty of equipment at your disposal, and provide a ready-made network of experts and some friendly camaraderie, too. Most gyms know how important it is to create programming that appeals to newcomers, so look for one with plenty of different beginner-level options, including weight lifting classes. (Believe me, no one—not even the biggest show-off—was born knowing what to do with all those weight machines. Everyone has to start at the beginning.)

Before joining, have a good long talk with yourself about what you like to do. Now, check out the gym at the time you think you are most likely to go: Is the stuff that appeals to you, like a Spin class or group weight lifting, available then? A place with a leisurely vibe at lunchtime can be a madhouse after work, so make sure the energy level appeals to you. Does the gym have trainers available to show you around initially

Best time of day to **Work Out:**
Late Afternoon

While the research is a bit controversial, some circadian rhythm experts say that in an ideal world, working out in the late afternoon is best for most people, both in terms of performance and attitude. And for all of you living in an ideal world, I'm very happy for you!

But for the rest of us, the best time to exercise is anytime we can fit it in and make it a happy activity. For me, that's the early a.m. For many people I know, it's in the evening. Whatever time slot you choose, stick with it—it will become a feel-good habit sooner than you think.

and for hire at an hourly rate (pretty standard in the industry), and are trainers also walking around from time to time, offering friendly pointers and encouragement? Do people seem to know each other, or are they anonymous?

These points may seem unimportant, but it helps to understand that there is a huge dropout level at gyms—about 20 to 30 percent per year, by some industry estimates. Often people say they lost their momentum early on and stopped going because it felt too impersonal, as if no one noticed whether they showed up or not. (That's probably why people who work out with a buddy—a spouse, friend, sister, neighbor, or co-worker—are more likely to stick with it.) Classes are also a great way to motivate yourself and to meet people.

LOOK FOR PEOPLE WHO ARE LIKE YOU. "There are many trainers and instructors who specialize in specific populations," Calabrese says, "from people with knee problems to cancer patients to those considering gastric bypass." It may turn out that a smaller gym—with fewer machines and a less-glitzy changing room—is actually more supportive. Philadelphia trainer Debra Mazda's ShapelyGirl gym, for example, specializes in plus-size women, because that's her expertise. "I weighed 325 pounds, and I was on every diet—I even had my jaws wired shut—and nothing worked. Then I said to myself, 'These people are exercising and thin,' and I thought, 'Let me try.' When I started to exercise, the weight began falling off me." Although Mazda has used exercise and healthy eating to maintain the same weight for 25 years, she remembers how

Make 1 Minute Count

Twice this week, I want you to do something very hard for you, but only for a minute. Some ideas: jumping rope, jumping up on a step, or bursting into a run from a walking pace. And no, my goal isn't to torture you. This extreme exertion forces you to breathe really hard, forcing more oxygen into your body.

My challenge move: _____

intimidating it was to begin working out. "So we'll start out with easier treadmill or exercise bike workouts," she says, "and when they want to start experimenting with classes, we make it easy for them to step back if they can only keep up for 10 minutes or so."

SET EASY-TO-MEASURE GOALS. While saying "I wanna lose 15 pounds and 2 inches off my tush" sounds superspecific, these aren't actually the best kinds of exercise goals, behavioral change experts say, because you really can't control how fast that happens. What works better are mini-goals that *are* completely in your control, like "I'll go to the gym after work at least three times this week." These are what the pros call process goals, rather than product goals, and they help you stay motivated because they are more easily met.

And in my practice, I've really become a big believer in the power of consistency. People who say, "I'm going to work out three times a week," and then really do it for a period of time, build confidence in their ability to stick with a program and can then move on to add new routines and tweak the intensity or up the number of sessions they do. In fact, I think people who can achieve consistency are better off than people who exercise very intensely occasionally, because that on-again, off-again approach is discouraging and can lead to soreness and injuries.

The conventional wisdom is that any exercise is better than none, but I think that's a little bit of a cop-out. Yes, I applaud any change and know it isn't easy. But at the same time, I have to be candid: The best guidelines—from those issued by the US Department of Health to those by the American College of Sports Medicine—are that you should exercise most days of the week, meaning at least 4 days, and that your routine should include anywhere from 20 to 60 minutes of cardio, as well as strength training twice a week and stretching.

Remember, this is an 8-week plan. And 56 days isn't an accidental number—some experts say that's how long it takes to build a healthy habit.

Write your goal for the first 4 weeks of the plan. Then revise them for the next 4 weeks.

CARDIO GOAL: **20 MINUTES, 4 DAYS A WEEK**

Days:

Type:

Minutes/Workout:

Please don't think that 20 minutes of cardio means you have to go charging off to do uphill sprints. A brisk walk counts if it gets your heart rate going. Not sure if you're walking fast enough? Rely on the trusty "perceived rate of exertion" measure: If you're working so hard you can only talk in one-word gasps, back off! That's too intense. And if you can converse or sing freely, step on it—you're not working hard enough. For now, you're looking a pace at which you can manage short sentences but that makes you feel you're a little winded. And feel free to take this in small doses: Two 10-minute sessions count just the same as one 20-minute one. If that feels easy—and you may well be in better shape than you think—increase the duration to 30 minutes and step up the intensity a bit.

WEIGHT GOAL: **2 DAYS A WEEK**

Days:

Type:

Time:

I love lifting weights, but my ideal day of heavy lifting involves swinging my kids around or hanging on some monkey bars. If you aren't a gym person (or at least not yet!), I encourage you to find ways to work strength training into your regular routine. Kids and pets offer plenty of opportunities for extra lifting. Many clients also like to use DVDs with free weights to get started. (Many people say they can't stay motivated working out with DVDs at home, but for others, it's a great way to work out—when no one but the cat is watching you, you don't have to be self-conscious!)

Don't know where to begin? Drop down and give me 20! Seriously, superbasic old-fashioned pushups, done from your knees or even against the wall to get started, are as effective as ever. Again, 20 at once is hard. So do as many as you can and then take a break. On days when I can't get to my usual workout, I do pushups . . . anywhere! I've done them in my office, in hotel rooms—even in the green room of a TV studio!

It's a great idea to start an exercise log—go to www.nutritiouslife.com for a food and exercise journal—and keep it for the full 8 weeks of the plan. That way, you can assess it each week to see if you're paying enough attention to strength, cardio, and stretching. Add your weekly challenge moves for bonus points!

Workout Plan 2

YOU'RE FIT, BUT YOUR ROUTINE HASN'T CHANGED MUCH

To me, one of the most wonderful things about staying fit is that it's a constant challenge. As soon as a new exercise gets too easy, I get to tweak it or bring it to the next level. A huge sense of personal power

My Boredom Buster

Seasoned exercisers are a little more vulnerable than other people to falling into mental ruts. No matter how devoted you are to your routine, pick one new thing to try each week—maybe on the weekend, when you have a little more time. Try a new class at the gym, ditch Pilates for a Spin class, check out a workout DVD from your library, dabble in some online classes (FitSugar and Gaiam offer some popular ones). Borrow your kid's scooter and take it for a spin! The point is to spend at least a little time each week finding something new to love about exercise.

comes from graduating from pushups on your knees to the real he-man variety, or realizing that the "challenging" pace on the rowing machine last week feels more comfortable now.

But some people don't like that. In fact, they fall into fitness ruts, jumping on the treadmill and covering the same distance at the same pace, month after month, even year after year. If you fall into this category, you may like to think you're getting fitter—and I hate to be the bearer of bad news here—but you're not. Are you fitter than a nonexerciser? You sure are, and good for you. I don't want to take any credit away from you for your discipline or diss your efforts in any way. But you're not gaining fitness, and chances are—depending on your age and what you do for a living—you're probably not even maintaining it.

The truth is that the only way to build fitness is to continually add novel movements. Building fitness requires making new demands on

Might As Well *Jump!*

If you're working out regularly, you're already part of the fitness elite. (Remember, groups like the American College of Sports Medicine estimate that 60 percent of Americans aren't exercising enough.) So, don't you think it's time to flex your muscles and get a little . . . swagger?

When athletes are boosting their conditioning level, they use moves called plyometrics—the kind of hard-core drills you might see football or soccer players do at practice. I'm not asking you to go out for the NFL, but if you already have a reasonable level of fitness, you'll benefit from some tough challenges. Even a few minutes of plyometrics a week can increase your fitness, build your bones, and protect you from injury. Sometimes called jump training, these moves can be done at home. Start by jumping up on a step, or try a deep squat, followed by a jump. (Start with a few sets of eight repetitions, and see how intensely your leg muscles feel it the next day!)

Besides the big jump in confidence, you'll also get more health benefits. The American Council on Exercise says high-intensity, power-based exercises are effective for burning a high number of calories in a short period of time. They also promote the anabolic hormones, such as HGH and IGF-1, that are responsible for muscle growth and can actually have an antiaging effect.

your body. As soon as it becomes accustomed to a workout, no matter how easy or how hard core, it stops being challenged. Your muscles are no longer stressed in response, and they aren't building.

"All in all, being active is the key to life," says Kathy Kaehler, celebrity trainer and creator of Sunday Set-Up. "Staying fit keeps you young. Keeping your workout fresh is the way to a lifetime of exercise."

I get it—I have a life, too (at least, most days I do). But the wonderful thing is that there are plenty of ways to continually ramp up your fitness level, without adding more time to your routine. That's important to me, too. I actually love long, leisurely workouts, but they don't fit into my schedule the way they did before I had kids. Honestly, I have to shoehorn as much as possible into my 30 to 40 precious minutes!

Back in the mid-1990s, a Japanese researcher named Izumi Tabata made a discovery that's invaluable to time-challenged people. While athletes had been using interval training—working much harder for very short spurts, then dropping down to less intense levels again—he and his team found that by using intervals, he could actually build fitness in much less time. The breakthrough discovery came from a bunch of mice. One group swam for long periods, and another group swam intensely for 20 seconds and then rested for 10 seconds, eight times. (See, I told you eight was a magic number!) And they were just as fast! Think of the beautiful time-saving math in that sentence: By working out for 4 minutes, they achieved the same fitness benefits as the mice that swam for much longer. You don't have to be a wet mouse to know that's a good deal.

You can put the Tabata concept to work in virtually any situation, explains Jennifer DiDonato, a personal trainer in the Detroit area. "Take crunches," she says. "Many people don't like counting the number of reps. Instead, you just do as many as you can for 20 seconds then rest for 10 seconds, eight times. After 4 minutes, you've done a complete—and intense—set of ab work." But be careful, she warns, that you don't go so fast that you lose proper form: "You don't want to injure yourself."

She also likes to program these 20-second intervals into treadmills and other exercise machines, or use a stopwatch with clients while walking. "When your body adapts to the challenge of your usual work-outs, your body could plateau." She says the Tabata method can offset that. "Just do something faster than what you're used to, to up the ante." The intervals "improve overall cardio efficiency and burn fat more efficiently," she says. "That doesn't mean you want to increase your entire workout by sprinting the whole time," DiDonato says. "The point is you want to hit all your heart zones a couple of times during a workout to improve our body's ability to burn more fat for fuel while at rest."

An American College of Sports Medicine study found that interval training for runners can increase heart stroke volume (the amount of blood it pumps with each heartbeat) by about 10 percent. Slower, sustained running has no effect on it.

Increasingly, researchers are finding that this concept really builds fitness, helps your heart, and burns calories. A study from McMaster University in Canada found that a 20-minute workout that consisted of a minute of intense riding on a stationary bike with a minute of rest, performed three times a week, improved cardiovascular measures just as much as an hour of biking at a slower pace did. This type of training, called HIT, for "high-intensity interval training," is becoming more and more popular, so look for classes in your area.

Write down your goals for the first week of the plan. Then revise them each week after that.

CARDIO GOAL

Days:

Type:

Minutes/Workout:

I'd like to see you strive for 45 minutes, at least four times a week, with some form of intervals—maybe even 4 minutes of Tabata intervals of situps or pushups!—built in.

WEIGHT GOAL

Days:

Type:

Reps/Workout:

If you've already got a regular weight routine you feel is adequate, don't mess with it too much, but do look for smaller ways to mix it up. Maybe you could stand to lift a little more. Pick at least three strength moves you want to improve.

Workout Plan 3

YOU'RE REALLY FIT. NOW MAKE YOUR WORKOUT HELP YOU DROP MORE WEIGHT

Because I've been lucky enough to work on nutrition plans with professional athletes, and because I've been accused of being a little—ahem!—*driven* in the fitness department myself, I know that being really fit takes a lot of time, energy, and commitment. And over the years, I've helped my clients get ready for everything from marathons to triathlons to mountain-climbing expeditions. I respect your goals, and it's not my job to tell you you're training too hard, especially if you're happy and injury free.

But it is up to me to suggest a few changes in order to maximize the power of the New You and Improved Diet. First, when was the last time you sized up your workout regimen for blind spots? Training for an event can—and should—involve escalating levels, but has your extra cycling squeezed out the yoga class that made your back feel better? Has your strength training gotten so much more interesting that you've sort of slacked off on cardio without realizing it? If you don't already have one, start an exercise log and keep it for the full 8 weeks of the plan. Assess it each week to see if you're paying enough attention to strength, cardio, and stretching. (I've made a column for exercise in the food journal on my Web site, www.nutritiouslife.com to make it easier, but many of my clients and friends love using workout apps.)

Consider a session or two with a trainer who specializes in your fitness routine or sport to get a technique checkup. Often, it's the shortcuts we take—usually without realizing it—that shave off a little effectiveness and also put us at a bigger risk for overuse injuries.

Write down your goals for the first week and then for each week after that.

CARDIO GOAL

Days:

Type:

Minutes/Workout:

I'd like to see you strive for 60 minutes, at least four times a week, with some form of intervals. And I'd like you to add something new: If you bike, try the rowing machine; if you use the elliptical, switch to the treadmill. You already know how to push the needle in terms of intensity, but the whole point of cross-training is to push your comfort zone in terms of variety.

WEIGHT GOAL

Days:

Type:

Reps/Workout:

Focus on your three weakest areas, and be honest. We all tend to lift the weights most where we're strongest and neglect where we're weakest, which is the perfect recipe for an injury. Maybe you can bench-press your weight—good for you. How strong is your back? Consider a session with a trainer who will give you objective feedback. Pick at least three areas you want to improve.

Keri's Eight Favorite
Foods for a Fitter You

In some ways, all foods are good workout foods. They all provide calories, which, of course, our body uses for energy. That said, nutritionists are learning more—with new research piling up every day—about what foods best support the demands of physical exertion with the goal of losing weight. Here are my eight favorite get-fit foods, based on that research and what's worked best for my clients over the years, along with what makes me feel like tearing it up on my morning run.

CHOCOLATE MILK When I'm in the gym, it makes me cringe to see so many people guzzling sugar-packed sports drinks after a healthy workout. While the Gatorades of the world have made billions convincing people that they need these overly sweetened drinks with electrolytes, the truth is that for most workouts (unless they're superintense or over an hour), there's no need. Chocolate milk is one of the best "recovery" drinks, especially after weight lifting. It's got protein—20 percent of which is whey protein, the same ingredient many people buy as a supplement. Plus it's hydrating and has calcium, some sodium, and just enough sugar to get your metabolism going. And a University of Texas at Austin study tested chocolate milk against both other sports drinks and plain old water, and it performed better. Over time, athletes who drank chocolate milk after a workout built more muscle and lost more fat. Don't forget to count it in your plan as a milk!

COCONUT WATER This product has gained popularity, and fans love it, especially in place of a sports drink (which is often recommended for rehydrating after an intense workout that lasts more than an hour). Coconut water has potassium and electrolytes, and because it's a natural product, right from inside a coconut, it doesn't have chemicals like a sports drink. (But always read the label, just to be sure.) Some research has shown coconut water hydrates just as well as a sports drink, and it quenches your thirst a bit better than plain old water. Coconut water tends to be a little more expensive than sports drinks and slightly lower in calories. Not everyone loves the flavor, but I do!

LEAFY GREENS A diet with plenty of leafy greens supports a strong skeleton. You already know about spinach, of course, but I think this is a good time to introduce you to the power of bok choy, collard greens, and kale. Leafy greens pack high levels of vitamin K, which aids in the production of proteins essential for bone health. I like to buy big bunches on the weekend, wash them, and keep them chopped and ready to go in zipper-lock bags in my crisper. That way, they're easy to toss into eggs, salads, soups, or stir-fries. Another bonus is that carotenoids in leafy greens have been proven to slow sarcopenia, the natural damage that occurs in our muscles as we age.

LOW-FAT RICOTTA I'm a big fan of cottage cheese, but not everyone is, and I've found that ricotta has a wider appeal, maybe because the texture is a little creamier. Ricotta is great for strength training. It's made from whey protein and also boasts beta-lactoglobulin, a protein some researchers have found helps muscles rebuild themselves. Protein is especially good to eat after weight training, and if you add a small amount of easily absorbed carbohydrate to your ricotta—perhaps half a banana, a teaspoon of honey, or some chopped-up apples—your muscles will absorb its protein benefits even faster.

QUINOA This tasty little grain has a rare quality: It's a perfect protein, with all eight essential amino acids, so it can help your body recover quickly from a workout. It's also lower in calories than many other grains. It isn't just a good carb; it's a great carb. Serve it as a side dish, flavored with broth, or as a main course with vegetables and leftover chicken.

RAISINS Sweet and super portable, these wrinkly little gems can be sprinkled into yogurt or cottage cheese, or you can just tear open one of those cute little red boxes and eat them plain. As with all dried fruit, it's important to be mindful of your portion—as the water evaporates, the sugar becomes more concentrated, and it's easy to overdo it and consume too many calories. But as a performance food, you can't beat 'em. One study compared the blood levels of insulin, lactic acid, and other key chemicals in cyclists who'd completed a long-distance ride after eating either raisins or a high-tech (and pricey) sports gel. Cyclists who'd eaten raisins performed just as well as those who'd eaten the manufactured good. Plus, raisins taste great!

TOMATOES Sliced in salads or simmering in a sauce, tomatoes seem to go with everything—no wonder they're the fourth most popular vegetable in the United States. They're loaded with lycopene, and researchers have found that the higher the serum level of this antioxidant found in people's blood, the lower the level of heart disease as well as other chronic illnesses. And unlike with some other vegetables, cooking actually increases tomatoes' nutritional power. Their high level of vitamin C helps your body better respond to stress. And if you've got knee pain or any signs of arthritis, don't worry about that old myth of foods from the nightshade family (that includes tomatoes and green peppers) making your symptoms worse. Some research has shown that people who eat lots of the foods popular in the Mediterranean (and you better believe that includes lots of tomato sauce!) actually suffer from less inflammation than others and even regain some physical function.

TUNA, IN CANS OR POUCHES While all protein foods help support the muscles you're building when you exercise, there's a reason tuna is such a favorite with bodybuilders. Packed in water, it's an incredible calorie bargain. And from a busy dieter's standpoint, it's easy to keep plenty of cans or pouches of it in the pantry. But tuna doesn't just have protein. It also contains lots of niacin and vitamins B_6 and B_{12}, plus selenium, a mineral that's an important antioxidant. For a delicious combo, toss some in a glass container with brown rice and bring it to work or the gym. And because I worry about the amount of mercury that's infiltrated so many fish, I like Wild Planet's Minimal Mercury canned tuna.

What Happens When You Don't Exercise

Looking at things strictly from a health perspective, it turns out that keeping active is actually more important than maintaining a healthy weight. (Being a registered dietitian, I don't always like admitting that, but it's true!) A growing body of evidence has shown that normal-weight couch potatoes are more vulnerable to all causes of death, but especially those due to heart disease, than are overweight people who exercise regularly. Among the biggest risks:

SEDENTARY WOMEN ARE MORE AT RISK FOR DIABETES

Women who don't exercise and who sit for long periods—that's most of us with desk jobs—are more likely to develop type 2 diabetes, according to researchers in the U.K. (The same doesn't seem to be true for men.)

THE NEW YOU! Some of the most impressive new studies have shown that a sedentary lifestyle—sitting most of the time—puts even regular exercisers at risk. Because we're focusing on small steps, and because the plan encourages you to make incremental changes that increase your activity level even if you don't go to the gym, you can get those health perks without wearing spandex. Start moving whenever you can.

YOU'LL BE AT RISK FOR OTHER HEALTH PROBLEMS, TOO

Again, the culprit, according to the American Institute of Cancer Research, isn't not exercising but rather the average 15.5 hours of sitting so many of us do each day. The large, idle muscles, researchers speculate, crank out biomarkers that up the odds for disease.

THE NEW YOU! Besides the incremental bits of activity and exercise you'll be adding each of the 8 weeks on the plan, the New You and Improved Diet contains plenty of produce, because a plant-based diet is one of the best-known ways to prevent cancer. More important, the types of produce I've included each and every day on the plan are specifically chosen for their high level of antioxidants, another proven weapon in your anticancer arsenal.

YOU'LL GET HEADACHES, ACHY KNEES, AND A SORE BACK

While people often groan about little aches and pains when they start an exercise routine, the truth is that not moving is what hurts us. Sedentary living has been linked to migraines and other headaches, joint pain, and even arthritis and back issues. You won't sleep as well at night or have as much energy in the day.

THE NEW YOU! A gradual increase of activity and exercise not only speeds weight loss and fends off serious disease, but also keeps your joints and bones moving better. People who exercise have fewer back injuries than those who don't. Exercisers also sleep better and have higher energy levels, which means they're happier and more productive at work.

Feel Sexy to Slim Down

It's not what I do,
but the way I do it.

—MAE WEST

L et's talk about sex. And whether that sentence made you think "Do we *have* to?" or "Thank God! I like sex! At least she isn't going to talk anymore about exercise or kale," the truth is that sex has much more of an impact on how well you do on the New You and Improved Diet and on your overall health than many people realize.

Yep, sex—or lack of it—may be sabotaging your diet. And simply rethinking a few things may allow you to turn it around, and make your

Feel Sexy to Slim Down:
HOW IT CONNECTS

Lots of times, clients will balk when I tell them this rule and ask that they take time to think about the quality of their sex life. Often they'll say, "Whoa! What's *that* got to do with my weight?" But the reality is, sex is intricately linked to well-being, for both women and men. A healthy sex life, with plenty of cuddles, boosts self-worth as well as oxytocin, a hormone that helps you manage stress (Rule No. 2) and sleep more soundly (Rule No. 7).
When you feel strong and sexy, you're more likely to take the time to baby yourself now and then (Rule No. 6). And when you eat well (Rule No. 1) and hydrate properly (Rule No. 3), you'll notice sex feels better, too.

sexuality one of your most powerful health and weight loss allies. I think that having a good, healthy sex life is so important that I've made it one of the eight pillars of my practice and a key component of the New You and Improved Diet.

That doesn't mean it's easy to talk about, though. Often, when I bring it up in early sessions with a client, she'll make a face and hold up her hand, as if begging me to stop. "Blechh," she might say. "How can I feel sexy? I'm fat." It's as if even mentioning sex somehow puts pressure on her to look so impossibly good that she'll run home and start dancing around the bedroom in high heels and a thong, to which I can only say . . . "No! No! No!"

To me, feeling good about your sexuality is a measure of health, not of how much you weigh or how you think you look in a bathing suit. It's not even about how often you have sex—some of the healthiest people I know, by the way, are in between relationships. So when I say "sex," please don't think I want you to race into dating, or to sleep with your current sweetie or spouse any more than you want to. I'm simply talking about taking such good care of this important aspect of yourself that when you look in the mirror, you say, "Wow—I am looking pretty darn good today!" (We'll get into the clinical side of it shortly.)

I want you to walk down the street feeling good about yourself, inside and out, and knowing that you have a right to be happy in every area of your life. If a client seems supersensitive to the word *sexy,* sometimes I'll switch to my clinical voice and instead use expressions like "positive body image." It's a sense of knowing that, of course, you are luscious and desirable. Of course, you are strong and healthy. And of course, you are as in control of your sexual nature as you are of how you eat, drink, work, and handle stress. Why shouldn't a diet help you function as well in the bedroom as you do in the kitchen, office, or gym? It's all part of who we are, and the sooner we can separate that feel-good sexual part of our personality from some twisted idea of what we're supposed to look like in lingerie, the happier we'll all be.

A poor body image positively haunts people, especially women today. I don't like to be melodramatic, but it is such a source of unhappiness. A majority of women perceive themselves to be overweight and are unhappy with their bodies. This includes plenty of women who aren't the least bit heavy. And the unhappier people are with their bodies, the more likely they are to eat poorly and to go on binges here or there. It's the women who feel most unhappy with themselves who are also the most likely to run crying into the arms of Ben & Jerry. One survey practically made me cry: It polled a random sampling of 300 young women and found that 97 percent had at least one cruel thought about their body every day, like "You're a fat pig" or "Your thighs are hideous." On average, these women reported 13 such nasty thoughts *per day.*

Not exactly the frame of mind to think of yourself as an untamed tigress in the bedroom, is it? A beaten dog is more like it! That kind of body bashing has taken a pretty big toll on our national libido. A study of 31,000 women, 18 and older, found that an incredible 43 percent reported at least some level of sexual problem. Among women ages 18 to

44, 10 percent have persistently low sexual desire; among older women, it's nearly 15 percent.

And in studies of women who are overweight, the numbers go up drastically. Researchers at Duke University have found that 30 percent of those who are overweight or obese struggle with sexual drive, desire, or performance—and very often, all three.

Men aren't immune, either. Many of my male clients have a level of ab shame that women can't even imagine. They think they're supposed to have the same six-packs they see airbrushed onto so many magazines, and that others expect that from them. When I tell them the hours of hard work male models have to put in to look like that, they're stunned.

And actually, this is one of the best parts of my job. That's because clients who come to see me with the "simple" goal of getting back into a size 6 dress or having a 32-inch waist just aren't aware of how profound a change healthy weight loss can be. So while they may never have been able to articulate a goal like "I want to feel better about my body so I can enjoy sex more," that's what happens. (I've made a lot of significant others very grateful, by the way!)

I hope you know that when I talk about sexual health, I'm not only talking about Saturday night, lace underwear, and scented candles. In fact, if there's one thing we're always learning about sex, it's that it means many things to many people. I was blown away by a recent study showing that most of us aren't even really sure what we mean by "sex," anyway. While virtually everyone agrees that good old-fashioned intercourse counts as "having sex," there is no consensus on whether

"Keri, what about alcohol and romance?"

I know lots of people like wining and dining before romance, and for many people, a drink is a really good way to get in the mood. (Studies have shown that having a drink or two really can help many women relax, get in the mood, and even enjoy sex more.) But be careful: In some men, alcohol consumption can interfere with performance. And for both men and women following the New You and Improved Diet, drinking too much will slow down your weight loss.

that's true of other types of sexual activity, even using your own hands. You have my permission to define sex any way you want. My job here is only to explain that it's good for you in so many ways, and it all boils down to making it easier for you to stay on track with the New You and Improved Diet. And no, it's not because sex burns calories. (It does, but not nearly as many as my clients think it should!)

I define "sex" as anything frisky, sweet, and satisfying—whether it's masturbating, sex with a spouse, a flirtation with the barista who makes your coffee every morning, or even a good old-fashioned foot rub. In fact, these kinds of incidental exchanges turn out to be enormously important: A recent study from the Kinsey Institute at Indiana University found that cuddling and caressing are more important ingredients than sex in being satisfied in a long-term relationship. This study even found something a little shocking: Frequent cuddling and kissing are bigger predictors of a man's happiness than a woman's! So much for sexual stereotypes, huh?

I'm not saying the New You and Improved Diet will give you some kind of Mae West/Angelina Jolie/George Clooney swagger, although that wouldn't be a terrible thing. But you will start to notice an improvement in your libido, a new respect and love for your body, and—thanks to all the wonderful deep breathing you're doing—a refreshingly calm and open way to see your sexual self. In fact, one of my favorite things is how having a more relaxed, open, and positive attitude about sex works together with the other seven rules: Nutrition, stress management, hydration, and exercise all support a sexier you. And a better sex life makes you more relaxed, less stressed, sleep more soundly . . . It's a wonderful cycle!

Here are some of the ways the other New You and Improved Diet rules intersect with sex.

EATING EMPOWERED SUPPORTS YOUR SEXUAL HEALTH. The nutritious foods you'll be eating on this plan will help your sex life in two very important ways. First, the more body fat a person has, the higher the level of a substance called sex hormone binding globulin, or SHBG. It binds to testosterone, a sex hormone both men and women need to have a healthy libido. The good news? Losing as little as 10 pounds has been shown to stimulate sex hormones, perking up sex drive.

Second, the healthy foods you'll be eating control both cholesterol and blood sugar levels, improving your blood flow. And while most people are aware that poor blood flow causes sexual problems for men, in the form of erectile problems, it also affects the amount of blood flowing to a woman's clitoris. And when your body is less responsive, it's only natural that you'll have less desire for sex.

MANAGING STRESS STRENGTHENS YOUR SEX LIFE. Chronic stress squelches sexual desire in both women and men, although scientists think it works a little differently in each. Researchers in the lab have found that stress changes levels of serum sex hormones in the blood, as well as catecholamines, the hormones produced by the adrenal glands, which are found on top of the kidneys. These include dopamine, norepinephrine, and epinephrine (formerly called adrenalin). In my own field research on this, though, I think it's much simpler: Stress makes me tired and unhappy, and therefore, not in the mood.

One thing I love about sex, though, is that it has the power to reverse the negative effects of stress. A study from Arizona State University tracked 58 middle-age women for 9 months and found that, for the most part, sex put them in a good mood well into the next day, and they reported their stress levels were lower as well. And here's a cool thing: The more positive their mood, the more likely they were to have sex

Best time of day to **Have Sex:**
Early!

So, mornings turn out to be the ideal time to have sex, and it's not why you think—although, yes, many men do wake up with erections every day. It turns out that for both men and women, oxytocin levels are at their peak when we first wake up, so pre-breakfast nookie is a good idea. (Of course, you're not going to hear me say there's a bad time of day for sex!)

with their partners. It's the very opposite of a vicious cycle, right? Sex and cuddling improve our mood and reduce our stress; improved mood and reduced stress increase the likelihood of future sex and physical affection.

The stress reduction that comes from sex isn't something we experience just in the moment, either—it's a health benefit we carry around with us in all areas of our lives. Scottish researchers, for example, measured the blood pressure of people during public-speaking exercises (considered by so many to be a major-league stress event) and found that speakers who had recently had intercourse were less stressed out than those who hadn't. (The study followed 46 men and women over a 2-week period.) Another Scottish study looked at a sample of more than 2,800 people and found that frequency of sexual activity didn't just correlate with sexual satisfaction but with other measures of health and well-being, as well.

One reason cuddling and sex are so healthy for women is due to Mother Nature's best hormone: oxytocin. Experts have nicknamed this one the "calm and connection hormone" because it soothes us and makes us feel closer to people around us, as well as acts as an antioxidant. It's made in the neurons of the pituitary gland and released in both men and women after orgasm—or even through cuddling or simply by holding hands. In pregnant women, it signals when to go into labor, and it controls milk flow during breastfeeding, and without it, women wouldn't bond so fiercely with their babies.

But we also create oxytocin just by giving someone a sign of trust. Researchers at Claremont Graduate University in California have found that when someone is given money, for example, that person feels trusted, triggering oxytocin, which then makes that person behave in a more trustworthy way. That makes them more inclined to trust people, and so on. No wonder the researchers also nicknamed oxytocin the "moral molecule"! (Some people also call it the "tend-and-befriend hormone.") And we don't even need to be face-to-face to have the oxytocin surges that come from human interactions. Researchers found that the good feeling from social connections even happens via Facebook and Twitter!

Here's how amazing oxytocin is: It works better than some medicines! Researchers at the University of North Carolina found that when couples spent just 10 minutes holding hands, oxytocin levels rose enough to significantly lower blood pressure. Psychologists at Northern Illinois University have recently found that higher levels of oxytocin are linked to socializing and keep us from feeling isolated, which could help prevent depression. And because women who breastfeed have lower risks of breast cancer, heart disease, stroke, high blood pressure, and diabetes, some researchers believe that their elevated levels of oxytocin may play a part in offering protection from these illnesses.

You actually don't need sex to stimulate this feel-good hormone—cuddling with pets will do the trick. The unconditional love of a furry friend might just be what you need. And hugs from good friends and family help, too.

Besides, single people are better off, health-wise, than those in unhappy marriages. Researchers have shown that people who are in relationships that are unsatisfying or full of conflict aren't just prone to anxiety and depression (you're shocked by that, I know!), but are also susceptible to physical issues, including heart disease, cancer, arthritis, and diabetes. Their wounds even heal more slowly!

Of course, oxytocin isn't the only chemical that's part of the sex equation. Canadian researchers have shown that levels of testosterone increase in both men and women after sex. They found that close physical intimacy, including cuddling, caused this rise, which seems to make women more open to sex—and to closer relationships—both long and short term.

Whatever chemicals are involved, a good sex life can make you happy. An Australian study tracked the sexual activity of 300 women and found that those who reported having a good sex life consistently scored higher on measures of anxiety, depression, cheerfulness, self-control, general health, and vitality.

EXERCISE IMPROVES YOUR SEXUAL RESPONSE. Besides helping you lose weight and balance stress, working out also boosts your sexual health and helps you achieve a steadier sex drive. Certainly, a big part of it is mental. Almost any form of exercise—even just adding more activity into your day or dancing around the living room now and then—will make you more conscious of your body, how it moves, how it feels, what it's capable of. And the more attention you pay to what your body is doing, the more likely you are to be attuned to what's going on with you sex-wise. Are you in the mood? Out of the mood? Staring at that guy on the elliptical more than you'd realized? Thinking that you haven't shaved your legs in ages? Those are all signs that you're just a little more conscious of your libido—an important barometer of sexual health.

I also think it's pretty natural that as you exercise and begin to notice changes in your body, even if it's just that you're able to lift slightly heavier weights or that you have a little more bounce in your step on the final lap of your daily walk, you'll carry some of that swagger with you into the bedroom!

But experts say that there's a strong physical component between physical activity and sex drive, too. Exercise that works the large muscle groups in the thighs and buttocks—walking, running, cycling, and yoga, for example, boosts the blood flow to your genital area and boosts your sexual desire.

Keri's Eight Favorite
Oh-So-Sensual Foods

Now that I've convinced you that you can definitely eat your way to a more satisfying sex life, experiment with these foods. Yes, they support your health (and weight loss) in many ways. But they also add a little spice in the sack.

CLOVES It's hard not to love this spice, which makes most of us think of steaming mugs of apple cider or heavenly holiday foods. But researchers at a university in India, a country where cloves have been used to treat male sexual dysfunction for centuries, found that clove extract "produced a significant and sustained increase in the sexual activity of normal male rats." (Around the world, it's also used to help with bad breath, and of course that's bound to make you a better kisser!) Cloves are one reason chai tastes so yummy, and I like to use powdered cloves in Mexican dishes, along with a little cumin and cinnamon.

GINGER Considered an old, reliable herbal remedy for nausea, ginger may also lower cholesterol and help prevent blood from clotting, suggest preliminary studies. Each of these effects may protect the blood vessels from blockage and the damaging effects of blockage such as atherosclerosis, which can lead to a heart attack or stroke. Anything that benefits the circulation and the heart can make good sex even better. And Canadian researchers say ginger is also linked to increased sexual desire. I think it's fun to serve pickled ginger, the kind you get with sushi, alongside fish or just about anything with a strong flavor—it's a real palate cleanser.

GINSENG A study at the University of Hawaii found that women who consumed a supplement containing ginseng not only saw a big increase in their libido in 4 weeks, but 68 percent of them also said their overall satisfaction with their sex life rose. Dabble in some of the yummy ginseng tea varieties at your natural foods store. One of my favorites is Ginseng Peppermint from the Republic of Tea. But be wary of energy

Fertility and Whole-Fat Dairy

Planning on getting pregnant soon? You might want to think about adding a daily whole-milk serving to the New You and Improved Diet. Research has linked the consumption of low-fat dairy products, which are an important part of my eating plan, to a type of infertility known as anovulatory infertility, in which the body fails to produce enough egg cells. Women who ate one serving of high-fat dairy food a day were 27 percent less likely to be infertile than women who avoided full-fat dairy foods, according to research from the Harvard School of Public Health. Swap out one serving of low fat for full fat.

drinks that claim to be ginseng laced—there's nothing sexy at all about the other chemicals and sugars that many of them contain.

OYSTERS While the legendary link between oysters and lovin' probably has more to do with the fact that they look a lot like female genitalia, oysters are a great source of protein. And they are rich in zinc, which is linked to increased libido, sexual performance, and, in men, better sperm production. But they are also just plain sexy to eat, especially slurping them raw, right off the half shell. For me, all they need is a little lemon and a touch of Tabasco sauce.

PEAS WITH AN EDIBLE POD Whether you choose snow peas or sugar snap peas, these sweet treats pack plenty of vitamin C, which helps your blood circulation. But as vegetables go, they also have an unexpected trick: While they contain just a little fat, it is omega-3 fat, with about 30 milligrams of alpha-linolenic acid (ALA) in a one-cup serving. And those ALAs are great for your heart and circulation, which in turn, is good for your sex life.

PUMPKIN SEEDS Known as *pepitos* south of the border, pumpkin seeds make great snacks and, like oysters, are high in zinc. They're also rich in omega-3s. I like to buy them still in the shell, and think they're a great boredom food—it's a way to pass the time in airports!

SAFFRON University of Guelph researchers say this subtle spice, which comes from the flowers of the crocus, can improve sexual performance. While it can be expensive, you need only a small amount of it for most recipes. Unsure how to prepare it? First, soak the threads in hot liquid for 15 minutes, and then add this saffron "tea" to soups, stews, or any grain, especially rice, quinoa, and barley.

WATERMELON Most of us eat this only in the summertime, but it's blessed with a high level of an amino acid called citrulline, which the body uses to make arginine, another amino acid. Arginine is related to vascular health, and in men, that can translate to healthier erections. But it's also been linked to increased libido in women, according to research from the University of Hawaii. It's sweet and hydrating and helps your libido—hard to say no to that, huh?

What Happens When You Don't Feel Sexy

Of course, I'm not saying people need sex to stay healthy. Some of the happiest, healthiest friends I have are single and love it. And there's tons of research that shows that nuns, for example, live longer than other women. I *am* saying, though, that when people don't feel sexy—when they don't like the way they look, or aren't paying close enough attention to their physical needs to know that they could use a cuddle, a massage, or even a little hand-holding—they're missing an inner spark of health, and something isn't quite right. It's like there's an important piston in your life that isn't firing. Here's what can happen:

IT'S LINKED TO DEPRESSION

For researchers, this link presents a bit of a chicken-and-egg problem. We know some 70 percent of people with depression also report a lower-than-normal libido. Does depression cause a low libido? Or does the low libido make people depressed? It almost doesn't matter, since experts say treating one so often helps the other.

THE NEW YOU! Not only will the meditation skills you're learning help you manage your moods (and in fact, mindfulness meditation has been shown to be as successful in treating depression as medication), but the combination of healthy foods and exercise will also foster a more positive outlook.

IT CAN ENCOURAGE A POOR BODY IMAGE AND BINGE EATING

If one of the reasons you're not as happy as you'd like to be with your sex life is that you have a lousy body image, that really concerns me. As common as body bashing is, it's also linked to binge eating, something that makes it really hard to stay on track with an eating plan. In more extreme cases, these distorted images of what we look like are linked to eating disorders such as anorexia and bulimia.

THE NEW YOU! By asking you to eat three carefully balanced meals each day, plus two snacks, I'm paying close attention to keeping your energy levels and blood sugar stable throughout the day, which is the best *physical* way to avoid binges. And your breathing practice—that mindfulness meditation—helps manage stress, another binge trigger.

Put Yourself First

Secure your own oxygen mask
before assisting others.

—EVERY AIRLINE I'VE EVER FLOWN

Whater I first talk to clients about this rule, I admit some of them balk. And I understand that the idea of pampering ourselves has a funny 1960s ring to it, all fluffy and superficial. People react as if all I'm talking about is bubble baths and manicures (not that there's anything wrong with either!).

But *pamper* is a word I use often and very deliberately, because it has an incredibly direct connection to how well—or how poorly—

Put Yourself First:
HOW IT CONNECTS

As obvious as it sounds, this is the rule that's often hardest for me to get across to new clients. Sometimes, I can almost see the words "take better care of yourself" bounce right off them in my office. Some think they are too busy; others, I suspect, think everyone else in their lives is more deserving of TLC than they are.

But I'm convinced no one can lose weight without mastering this basic idea of pampering. Usually, they've gained weight over the years because they translate the words "be good to yourself—you deserve it" into "splurge" foods that aren't good for them. At all. So without putting yourself first (Rule No. 6), it's practically impossible to eat well (Rule No. 1), because you'll constantly "treat" yourself with foods that sabotage your health goals instead of support them. A saner approach to self-care also makes it possible for you to manage stress better (Rule No. 2) and to sleep more deeply (Rule No. 7). Plus it can transform your relationship with exercise (Rule No. 4). Once you get the true meaning of the word *pamper,* you'll no longer head to the gym for stern punishment but find your way to workouts that both energize and calm you, flooding your brain with those feel-good hormones.

people do on the New You and Improved Diet. "Oh right," you're thinking. "Now she's going to tell me facials help you lose weight." And you know what? Pampering yourself—whether that means a gooey green facial mask, a day on the golf course, or sneaking off to see a movie on a weekday afternoon—*will* help you get back into your favorite jeans.

Here's why: You're not reading this book by accident. There are some very real reasons you may weigh more than you wanted to, and if I were to take you back through the years and years you've been cementing your eating habits, I bet I could build quite a case for all the times you believe you pampered yourself with food. You probably ate cakes and cookies as a treat when you were a kid; maybe your mom would joke about spoiling you with extra helpings of creamy tuna-noodle casserole. And as you grew up, you probably set up a system of rewards based on food. Of course, all those choices probably made you feel really good, at least while you were chewing and swallowing. But if you're like most people who come to see me, that good feeling didn't ever last very long. Pretty quickly, I bet, it was replaced with distress, unhappiness, and that weird kind of regret that only comes from overeating. Although the eating started out as a way to

Sunscreen, Self-Care, and Vitamin D

Whether I'm running outdoors, playing in the park with my kids, or just sitting in the sun reading, I consider being outdoors the ultimate "me time." And to make it even more relaxing, I'm really careful about protecting my skin from the sun. For a long time, this was a simple no-brainer, right? Sun exposure causes skin cancer and wrinkles, and besides, sunburns hurt!

But as recommendations and research about vitamin D continue to evolve—and as we learn more about some of the potentially scary ingredients used in many sunscreens—it's gotten more complex.

First off, we do need more vitamin D, although how much more has been a major source of controversy in the last decade. Essential for bone health, immune function, cancer prevention, and yes, weight control, we get this fat-soluble vitamin in dairy, fatty fish, cod liver oil, eggs, and fortified foods such as orange juice and breakfast cereals. But we can also make it ourselves from the sun. There are no exact recommendations yet, but a suggested range is anywhere from 5 to 30 minutes of sun exposure to the face, arms, back, or legs two or three times per week. But how fair your skin is, how far north of the equator you live, cloud cover, and the time of year all play a role.

For now, I'm sticking to the recommendations from the American Academy of Dermatology and wearing sunscreen everyday. It suggests products with both UVA and UVB protection, with an SPF of 30 or greater. To choose the ones with the least troublesome chemicals, I like to check in with the Environmental Working Group (ewg.org), which constantly updates its database and rates more than 1,800 brands.

"Keri, what about indulgent foods? I still want them!"

While most people on the New You and Improved Diet are constantly surprised (not to mention thrilled!) that they don't think much about "cheating," some people do struggle with these cravings, often in the form of an ice-cream spoon or a pasta fork. (Typically, these kinds of "gotta have it—now!" foods are very high in both carbs and fats.)

What's funny, though, is that the result often isn't what you'd expect. A new study tracked 160 women, checking their moods six times a day over a 10-day period. Surprisingly, even though the women described the meals they ate in restaurants in that time frame as indulgent, the meals tended to be followed by a negative mood. But the meals

(continued)

soothe you, it morphed into something kind of self-destructive.

As the years go by, these habits become more and more ingrained. The definition of a "good" night even gets a little warped. When you should be craving a nutritious, comforting meal, a calm evening, and a good night's sleep, you stuff yourself with four slices of pizza and a sleeve of Oreos, then watch 3 hours of crime dramas on TV, and get 6 hours of shut-eye before the alarm goes off—then you jump back on the merry-go-round the next day.

And over the years, perhaps you've grown so comfortable with these distortions that it's completely taken over your vocabulary. "I wanted to treat myself," a client will tell me, "so I ordered Belgian waffles *and* French toast." Or, "I work so hard, and I just finished a huge project at work, so I rewarded myself with a Never Ending Pasta Bowl."

Yes, I'll respond. You're 100 percent right. You *do* deserve a reward for how hard you work. Extraordinary efforts merit a treat. But that perk should be something that makes you feel good, not guilty. And if you eat something that makes you gain weight and then beat yourself up, where exactly does the feeling good part come in? It's like deciding to spend your vacation at a prison and then complaining because there are bars on the windows! Until you can learn to truly care for yourself, following Rule No. 1—eating well—will be very difficult, and losing weight will be much harder than it has to be.

So, you may not think of yourself as someone with a pampering deficit. But when I see someone who is overweight, or who tells me she's not in good control of what, when, or how much she eats, or who complains of too much stress or of seldom getting enough sleep, I know I am looking at a person who needs a little Pampering 101.

Sometimes my clients may not see themselves as being on the brink of burnout, but they are. And while most people use the term to talk about a professional problem, I know burnout is much bigger: Often, these people are diet and health burnouts, too. They've started, and stalled, on so many diets, exercise routines, and various self-improvements plans that they're exhausted. Many will confess to me—sometimes in tears—that they just don't believe anything can help.

That's where Rule No. 6 comes in: first, to help you learn to recognize those signs and symptoms of burnout, and second, to pamper yourself with things that really make you feel good. Think of them as nonfood rewards. Don't worry, I won't insist you get a $100 massage or head off to a luxurious spa. (But if you go, please take me along!)

I mean the little feel-good gifts we can give ourselves all day long to remind ourselves that we're doing a great job.

(continued)
they prepared and ate at home—which were healthier than what they ordered when dining out—produced many more upbeat moods. And the better their mood, the more likely the women were to make their next meal a healthy one, too.

Recognize that, ultimately, eating healthy foods makes you feel indulged. And eating indulgent foods makes you feel . . . abused!

If you've got a serious need to "spoil" yourself with a hot-fudge sundae—go for it! If it really scratches the itch and genuinely produces a feeling of pampering, good for you! But if it doesn't, you've learned something that will really help you in your weight-loss journey. Make a note in your food journal, and move on.

Remember, every meal is Monday morning—a clean slate and a chance to start over.

Drinking a glass of ice water out of your prettiest wine glass. Taking 10 extra minutes at the gym for a deep stretch. Curling up for a nap on a Saturday afternoon. These are all little presents we give ourselves, and they're the building blocks of true self-esteem. And yet, it's stunning to me how many people just don't get that they deserve to do this. Trust me—you *are* worth it.

And while I hate to stereotype, because I do believe this kind of self-neglect is almost an epidemic, I can safely say that women seem to run at a greater pampering deficit than men. I see it in myself. You try telling my kids that I need a break! They're kids, and when they're hungry, tired, or ready to run laps around me on the playground, they want to do it now! Clients, too, have a right to expect the best of me throughout the day and sometimes into the evening. And I pride myself on being there for my friends and family.

So, at the end of some days, I feel like there just isn't anything left over for me. I bet you can relate: I feel deflated, tired, and not at all myself. If it goes on for too long, I eventually get grouchy. To snap myself out of those mini-funks, I think about the wisdom you hear on every single airplane flight: Secure your own oxygen mask before assisting others.

Try More Nutrition on Your Skin

By now, you know what a firm believer I am in eating plenty of nutrients, and especially those in the antioxidant family, including vitamins A, C, and E.

But they work from the outside in, too. You can buy skin care products that provide these get-gorgeous nutrients, but I think it's fun to make these recipes on your own! Vitamin A, including chemicals in the retinol family, keeps skin looking younger by encouraging rapid cell turnover. Topical vitamin C has been proved to help collagen, a protein that keeps skin smooth and supple and repair itself more efficiently. And vitamin E is known to protect the skin from sun damage. There are plenty of other phytonutrient powerhouses that do wonders when applied topically, including ferulic acid (found in fennel, coffee, and apples), elegiac acid (found in many berries) and papain (derived from papayas).

Drugstore shelves are loaded with these products, and more arrive every day. Experiment, and see if you don't notice an improvement soon.

It always sounds just a little selfish to me. But it isn't. If I'm worn out and resentful, I'm not a good mom, a good mentor, a good daughter, or even a good boss.

For me, strapping on my own oxygen mask requires some very basic steps:

• I check my HQ. Have I eaten recently, and if so, what? What's missing? A protein serving? Did I skip a meal by accident? (I know, it almost never happens to me either, but I do like to check.) This supports Rule No. 1.

• Am I thirsty? I'll go ahead and make myself a mug of herbal tea to sip anyway. A cup of tea always makes me feel better. This supports Rule No. 3.

• Am I breathing? I breathe deeply, even if it's just for 2 or 3 minutes—that's usually enough for me to notice my shoulders are hunched up by my ears. And of course, this supports Rule No. 2—see the way the New You and Improved Diet rules all work together here?

• What have I done for *me* lately? I play back the last 24 hours and look for loving things I've done for myself. Have I used that fragrant lavender hand cream I bought? Flipped through a magazine for fun, not work? Called a friend? Made a plan for the weekend? Looked at some family photos? If it's been more than 24 hours since I did something a little pampering, I try to reward myself right then. If I can, I'll run myself a bath. (Go ahead, laugh at me and my bubble baths. They're truly thera-peutic!) Maybe I'll take a few minutes to listen to a favorite song on my iPhone. You get the idea: Food feeds my body, but these little acts of being gentle with myself actually feed my soul.

The Lost Art of Self-Care

Making those tender gestures a habit doesn't happen overnight. It takes practice and a steady commitment to taking care of yourself in all kinds of ways. But it's worth it, and pays off not just in greater weight loss but also in better health.

While I happen to love the word *pampering* (seriously, it makes me picture myself in a white terry cloth robe, relaxing on a chaise longue somewhere), scientists refer to it as "self-care." And because it is so mysterious and important, they study self-care—a lot!

For example, it's been well established that people in the "helping" professions—doctors, nurses, social workers, and *ahem*, nutritionists—tend to be very focused on patients and clients, often at their own expense. The result is burnout, which the experts define as a personal and professional syndrome that involves depersonalization, emotional exhaustion, and a sense of never really accomplishing anything. (Seriously, more than 7,000 medical studies have focused on the problem—that's how widespread it is!)

Of course, we all feel that way sometimes. But when that kind of self-neglect and empty feeling becomes chronic, people start to get a little reckless—those are the times when they're most likely to overdo it with food, alcohol, or both. "It was a 10 taco night," I remember one client telling me ruefully. "I have to learn that no matter how much I want to believe it in the moment, sour cream and extra cheese are not my friends anymore."

What protects people against that kind of burnout, these researchers find, are self-care skills, which is the psychological jargon for knowing

Be as Fussy about Your Skin
as You Are about Food!

In the same way I encourage my clients to read the labels on the food products they buy, I'd like you to start being just as fussy about skin care products.

Americans are nuts about antibacterials, for example. On the surface, that seems great—they slow the spread of colds, flu, and other illnesses. But some of the chemicals they contain are concerning. Triclosan, a common antibacterial chemical used in soaps, lotions, and even some toothpastes for at least 40 years, is hazardous. (Scarily, it's found in the urine of about 75 percent of Americans.)

So when I'm buying moisturizers and cleansers, I look for products that are free of:

- Parabens
- Mineral oil
- Phthalates
- Formaldehyde

when it's time to shut out the world, make a cup of tea, or coddle yourself with a favorite feel-good movie. Most encouraging, these researchers—who have also discovered that a good set of self-care skills improves the prognosis of people with everything from diabetes to cold sores to cancer—have demonstrated that such skills absolutely *can* be learned.

So school starts right now. Each day, beginning in the fourth week, on the New You and Improved Diet, I'm going to ask you to do something exceptionally nice for yourself—a deliberate pampering, private moment when you treat yourself to something special.

Keri's Eight Favorite
Pampering Foods

Eating well makes everything in the body function well, and that's bound to lead to a pampered feeling. In fact, it will give you an all-over cared-for, queen-for-a-day feeling, not to mention a beauty boost. (Yep, preventing burnout makes us look better!) On the New You and Improved Diet, don't be surprised if you get as many compliments about your skin, hair, or sparkling eyes as you do about your waist. (And I bet you'll notice your fingernails get stronger, too!)

These eight foods are especially powerful, and will do wonders for your skin, hair, and nails—as well as make you feel downright spoiled:

BRAZIL NUTS These nuts, which grow on very large trees in the Amazon region, are far and away one of the best sources of selenium, a mineral that's attracted a lot of attention in cancer research. For one thing, experts have discovered that the incidence of non-melanoma skin cancer is significantly higher in areas of the United States with low soil-selenium content. Other research has found that a selenium supplement significantly reduced the occurrence of and death from total cancers. And Brazil nuts are just a little bit more exotic than the usual almonds, walnuts, and peanuts. Try using them in pesto for a nice change of pace.

COCONUT I love this tropical wonder in all forms, as well as in a good piña colada every now and again. Coconut is said to improve the body's ability to absorb calcium and magnesium, minerals we need to keep our teeth strong and healthy. Bonus: Coconut's medium-chain triglycerides help burn fat. Spread two teaspoons of coconut butter on a high-fiber cracker for a delicious snack. (I use it as a moisturizer, too, right out of the jar.)

FIGS Women have been smearing fig products on their skin since biblical times, and I can't blame them—this fruit smells and tastes heavenly. And it's also packed with powerful antioxidants, which fight the effects of aging. Researchers have found that eating just a handful of dried figs increased people's antioxidant plasma level for 4 hours (much longer than many foods), and that was enough to offset the oxidative damage done by a carbonated soft drink! Thread them on a skewer and grill them for a nice treat, or serve them with thin slices of cheese.

HONEY Think of this as nature's antibacterial agent. When used on your skin, this beauty food is good for treating acne and reducing redness, and it's been proved to help skin heal more quickly. It's also a natural humectant, which means it keeps all that water you're drinking in the right places. A recent Welsh study of 665 people found that those who ate honey regularly were healthier than those who didn't, and had lower mortality rates over a 25-year period. While I think honey makes a nice addition to yogurt and cottage cheese, act like a kid again and spread a teaspoon on a slice of toast—it's as good as you remember!

LOBSTER These funny-looking ocean creatures are a terrific source of vitamin B_{12} and zinc, which help keep skin looking great. Too little zinc can cause hair loss and skin problems, while adequate amounts support faster wound healing and overall skin integrity. Hate the idea of cooking them yourself? Look for frozen lobster tails, especially for recipes like soups, stews, paella, and lobster salads. No one will know!

MUSHROOMS While brightly colored vegetables get much more of the research attention, fungi are emerging as nutritional all-stars. They've got B_6, folate, niacin, riboflavin, iron, potassium, and selenium. Once you start dabbling in 'shrooms, you'll be amazed at the variety—there are more than 35,000 kinds, many of them deadly. Try the woodsy maitake or hen-of-the-woods, melt-in-your-mouth oyster mushrooms, or the more strongly flavored shiitake. In ancient times, Chinese women ate them for a smooth complexion, and you'll find mushroom extracts in many high-end beauty products. You can buy presliced mushrooms in the produce aisle, to save you from washing, drying, and slicing them, though they're a little pricier.

PAPAYAS Another tropical treat, these bright orange fruits contain vitamins A, C, and E and papain, a digestive enzyme that is a mild exfoliant. When you eat papayas, these chemical compounds don't just help your skin look better—they're also good for your eyes, heart, and immune system. Vitamin C is vital for skin, but vitamin E is also essential, and an important way the body wards off sun damage such as age spots and wrinkles. Papayas are wonderful fresh, and dried papayas are as sweet as candy—and, in small amounts, naturally slimming!

ROSEMARY It's one of my favorite smells, and I love that it's sneaking into almost as many beauty products these days as it is into recipes. Whether we use it to season foods or topically, the fragrant oils stimulate circulation and act as an anti-irritant. I usually have a bottle of essential rosemary oil at work, and I'll sometimes put a few drops on a cotton ball and sniff. It doesn't just make you prettier; it's also a proven memory booster.

Best time of day to **Pamper Yourself:**
Late in the Evening

OK, there certainly isn't a bad time to treat yourself like royalty. But many people find it especially rewarding to save those special treats for the end of a long day. Truly pampering treats are relaxing and ease the transition from workday to bedtime. Listen to your favorite music. Spend a few minutes leisurely combing your hair. Find a pampering ritual and make it your own. My thing is coconut butter. I love to rub it on my feet, hands, knees, and elbows before bedtime—the smell is comforting and exotic at the same time, and the rich, creamy sensation on my skin makes me feel like a million bucks.

What Happens When You Skimp on "Me" Time

Researchers have found that certain types of people struggle more with self-care—and those taking care of others are the least likely to care for themselves. While anyone can run into occasional self-neglect ruts—most new moms have that zombie look, for example, and every accountant I've ever met looks pretty worn down by April 15—it can get to be a real problem. Here's what can go wrong:

YOU GO NUTS WITH A FOOD THAT SEEMS SOOTHING BUT REALLY ISN'T

Health researchers have found a persistent connection between poor self-care, low self-esteem, and binge eating. When you're neglecting yourself, certain foods start to seem nurturing. And whether you're drawn to the sweet comfort foods (ice cream comes to mind!) or the savory (mac 'n' cheese and gooey baked ziti), these foods aren't pampering. They're a guilt-a-thon waiting to get you.

THE NEW YOU! Between keeping a close eye on your HQ and taking plenty of deep breaths during the day, you'll notice a big improvement in your ability to know when you need to take a little time-out for yourself (cat video on YouTube, anyone?) rather than turning to a food that will sabotage your hard work.

YOU GET BLUE AND WANT TO GIVE UP

Researchers have found that for people with chronic health issues, whether it's diabetes, heart disease, or obesity, poor self-care makes focusing on routine health-management tasks harder. And in a kind of relentless circle, that makes health problems worse and it becomes common for depression to set in. The depression, then, makes caring for yourself even tougher.

THE NEW YOU! Because I am asking you to do small pampering things on a daily basis, and combining them with other health-building rules, you're less likely to get caught in this kind of slide. Just as negative results build on each other and start to snowball, so do positive ones!

Always Sleep Alone

Sleep is the best meditation.

—DALAI LAMA

sk anyone who knows me: When I have slept, I feel like I can conquer the world; when I haven't, I am cranky. I'm such an active person that when it's time for me to wind down—around 10 p.m.—I do it in a hurry. And I enjoy every minute of it.

Following Rule No. 7 will help you lose weight. A lot more weight. A team of sleep scientists at the University of Arizona in Tucson studied 245 overweight women, and found that sleeping 7 hours or more per night increased the likelihood that the women would lose weight, and keep it off, by 33 percent.

To me, sleep is almost as delicious as food. I love that feeling of climbing into bed and settling back against the pillow. And the early

Always Sleep Alone:
HOW IT CONNECTS

At this point, researchers have firmly established that getting enough sleep is key in weight management, so, of course, this supports Rule No. 1. Less well known, though, is the key role sleep plays in helping you bounce back from stress (Rule No. 2) And there's a wonderful yin-and-yang between sleep and exercise: The more sleep you get, the more effective your workouts (Rule No. 4). (In fact, many athletes routinely sleep more than the recommended 7 to 9 hours, because it's been shown to improve their performance.) And the more you exercise, the better you'll sleep!

morning, after a solid night's sleep, is just as luscious. When I wake up at 5:30 or so (this happens naturally for me—I don't even need to set an alarm), it's my favorite time of day. The world feels more peaceful, and the next 24 hours seem so full of possibility: Running through the early-morning streets of New York City is an amazing way to start the day!

But of all of my eight rules, this is the one I'm most likely to cheat on. I've been guilty of convincing myself (for short periods, anyway) that I really can get by on just 4 or 5 hours a night. And it works, at least for a few days. But then it catches up with me and turns into a kind of a nightmare. I get grouchy. I can't focus. And I find myself wanting to drink too much coffee or eat too much sugar to get my energy back. So I force myself to turn in early or take an afternoon nap on a weekend, and I feel my world shift back into balance.

I know many people share my struggle. That includes people who want to sleep but can't. People who fall asleep easily but wake up frequently. People who hate the idea of going to bed because there's too much fun to be had. And people who simply have so many things jammed into their day that adequate sleep isn't an option. (I have clients and friends who routinely send me e-mails at 3 a.m., and it makes me cry as much as if they were eating Doritos regularly for breakfast! I can't even imagine how ferocious and deranged I would be if I tried to do a 90-hour workweek even once, let alone week after week!)

Whatever your struggle with sleep, I'm here to tell you that this rule—always sleep alone—is absolutely critical to your weight loss results. And no, I don't want you to send your spouse or significant other to the couch or guest room! I mean banishing all of your electronics—your phone, your iPad, and your TV. Think of your bed as the perfect place for sleep, and of course, for sex! But everything else belongs outside the Inner Sanctum. This one is a struggle for me—I do love my iPhone!—but honestly, having a random text or e-mail chime startle me just as I'm about to drift off isn't worth it. I remind myself: "Keri, you're off duty! It's OK to be unplugged for 8 hours!"

Trust me, sleeping alone will make your weight loss easier. In the past decade, researchers have made very clear connections between weight gain and sleep habits: The less people sleep, the more they weigh.

In fact, some researchers believe that America's rising obesity rates may be closely linked to falling sleep levels. In the past 40 years, report University of Chicago researchers, American adults have whittled their average sleep time *a lot*. In 1960, US adults slept about 8.5 hours a night. But by 2002, that average had fallen to less than 7 hours a night, which means we are sleeping something like 550 fewer hours per year. The researchers found that the problem is even more extreme among young adults: The proportion of young adults sleeping less than 7 hours a night increased from 15.6 percent to 37.1 percent. And fewer than one out of four young adults now gets an average of at least 8 hours each night.

The researchers then linked those sleep decreases to increases in typical body weights and found a scary correlation. Back in 1960, when we all slept more, just one out of four adults was overweight, and only one in nine was considered obese. Currently, government statistics show that two out of three American adults are overweight, and one in three is actually obese.

The research demonstrated that partial sleep deprivation screwed up the levels of hormones that circulate in the bloodstream and regulate hunger, causing an increase in appetite. Worse, it caused cravings for calorie-dense, high-carbohydrate foods. Scientists studied 12 volunteers—all healthy young men—and found that when they slept only 4 hours a night for two nights, levels of leptin—the hormone that tells your body to stop, that it's had enough to eat—dropped by 18 percent. And levels of ghrelin—the hormone that says, "Keep going, eat more!"—jumped by 28 percent. And keep in mind, it didn't take weeks for that to happen; it just took

"Keri, why do my dreams change throughout the month?"

Sleep researchers at McGill University in Canada tracked the sleep of eight young women and found that while most aspects of the sleep cycle stayed the same throughout the month, there was a "modest but significant change in REM cycles." Other studies have suggested that it has to do with fluctuating body temperature: When women are premenstrual, we tend to dream more vividly, and also to remember our dreams more, than at other times throughout the month.

two nights. When I hear new moms saying, "I don't know why I can't lose this pregnancy weight," I understand why. Some experts estimate that a new baby typically results in 400 to 750 hours of lost sleep for parents in the first two years—no wonder the weight won't budge!

Additional research, from the University of Wisconsin and Stanford University, found that those who slept 7.7 hours or less per evening were more likely to be heavy. And since those early studies, which initially made big headlines back in 2004, evidence has continued to pile up, making an even stronger connection between too few z's and too many pounds. A recent analysis from Case Western Reserve Medical School followed more than 68,000 women for 16 years and found that those who slept 7 hours or less gained more weight and were more likely to be obese.

And a study from Columbia University found that women eat, on average, 329 more calories per day when they're sleep-deprived than when they're well rested. Considering that, typically, an average woman—about 5 feet 4 inches—with a relatively sedentary job needs to eat somewhere between 1,200 and 1,500 calories a day to maintain her weight, 329 extra is more than most women can afford.

Nor does it help that the kinds of snacks people hunt for when they're zonked often come in the form of the junkiest kind of carbs I can think of (anyone who has ever gnawed on an old greasy danish knows what I'm talking about). Then, they often get washed down with coffee or soda. And while those may help millions of sleep-deprived people get through the afternoon without looking like zombies, there's a price to be paid when the lights go out. Instead of dreaming about a beach vacation, people toss and turn.

Something else that's nice, and further proof of the wonderful ways these eight rules reinforce one another? Weight loss may help you sleep more deeply. That's because people who are overweight or obese have a higher incidence of something called sleep apnea. This disorder—most commonly found in men until age 50, when it turns into an equal-opportunity health risk—is tricky to diagnose, because so many people have it and don't realize it. Sleep apnea causes them to sleep fitfully and wake up frequently during the night, so they're not really sleeping deeply. (If you're the kind of person who sleeps 9 hours a night but still feels wiped out, *please* ask your doctor about this. The National Sleep Foundation says 18 million Americans have it.) While an estimated 70 percent of obese people have sleep apnea, there are many other risk factors. For example, Chinese women and African American women are more at risk.

How Sleep Works

The study of sleep, like that of nutrition, is relatively new. In fact, it was only in the mid-1950s that researchers were able to identify the different cycles of sleep, such as rapid eye movement (REM), and the link between REM sleep and dreaming.

Until then, most experts thought of sleep as very passive. Now, researchers know that our brains are very active during sleep, and in many different ways, and that it affects our daily functioning—including body weight. I like the way the National Institute of Neurological Disorders and Stroke (NINDS) explains it:

> Nerve-signaling chemicals called *neurotransmitters* control whether we are asleep or awake. Neurons in the brainstem, which connects the brain with the spinal cord, produce neurotransmitters such as serotonin and norepinephrine that keep some parts of the brain active while we are awake. Other neurons at the base of the brain begin signaling when we fall asleep. These neurons appear to "switch off" the signals that keep us awake. Research also suggests that a chemical called adenosine builds up in our blood while we are awake and causes drowsiness. This chemical gradually breaks down while we sleep.

Then, even though falling asleep feels instantaneous to us, these experts go on to say we typically pass through five phases of sleep—stages 1, 2, 3, and 4 and REM sleep—in cycles that repeat over and over throughout the evening. Most people spend almost 50 percent of their overall sleep in stage 2; about 20 percent in REM sleep, when most dreaming happens; and the remaining 30 percent in the other stages. Babies, on the other hand, spend about half of their total sleep time in REM land. (Here's another fun fact to amaze your friends: Elephants sleep standing up, except in REM sleep, when they lie down. No idea if they're dreaming, but at least they're more comfortable!)

Stage 1 is the light sleep, the kind that's so easy to drift in and out of that we often aren't even aware that we've been asleep. Our eyes move

Your Sleep Hygiene Checklist

What's your bedtime ritual? For me, it's using a favorite hand cream, listening to soothing music, and sipping chamomile tea as I organize my things (and the kids' stuff) for the next day. Take a moment to write down three to five things you will try to do consistently each night to ease your way toward a good night's sleep, and keep this list handy so you remember to wind down each night. Also, don't forget to give yourself a bed time!

very slowly and our muscle activity slows, but we can still wake up very easily if the phone rings or if someone knocks on the door. It's also the stage of sleep that often causes that weird bedtime sensation of falling, when we jerk ourselves awake. In stage 2 sleep, neurological experts say, our eye movements stop. Brain waves, caused by electrical activity, slow down, but there are also occasional bursts of rapid waves called sleep spindles—the intense electrical activity that makes the dramatic-looking hills and valleys you see in all those EEG readings on medical shows on TV. Both stage 1 and stage 2 are called light sleep—often, when we wake up, we aren't even sure we've been asleep.

In stages 3 and 4, which is what the pros call deep sleep, brain waves slow even further. Our eyes don't move, and there's no muscle activity. When we wake up from this kind of sleep, we're groggy and out of it, often for several minutes.

These four stages are called non–rapid eye movement sleep (NREM), and no one

"Keri, can certain foods make me dream?"

For years, I dismissed talk of dream foods as an old wives' tale. But if you're looking to have a more active dream life, you might try cheese: There is at least a little evidence that the peptides produced in milk might help. Cow's milk contains opioid peptides, including casomorphin, which has an effect comparable to that of morphine. (And that's why babies sleep so long when they have milk in their tummies.)

really knows why we need these stages of sleep, reports Medscape. One theory, though, is energy related: Because our bodies are making a much lower metabolic demand during sleep, it's a time for glycogen stores to be replenished in the brain.

Usually about 70 to 90 minutes after we fall asleep, we slip into REM sleep, when most dreams occur. REM sleep is essential to learning—which is one reason babies may need so much more of it than adults—and to problem solving. Our breathing becomes rapid, irregular, and shallow. Our eyes jerk around, and our heart rate and blood pressure go up. Men sometimes get erections. (In fact, some research has even found links between apnea, a sleep disorder, and erectile dysfunction. The theory is that those with sleep apnea have less REM sleep and, therefore, fewer nighttime erections.)

While a complete sleep cycle takes 90 to 110 minutes, the first sleep cycles each night contain shorter REM periods and longer periods of deep sleep. Then, as the night moves on, REM sleep periods get longer. The amount of deeper sleep we're getting declines. By morning, practically all of our sleep time is in stages 1, 2, and REM, according to NINDS.

Of course, while our brain is doing all this, other parts of our body have their own agenda. During sleep, our bodies crank out plenty of hormones, including growth hormones, which help kids grow and adults repair cells and tissues. Other hormones help fight off infections and boost our immune system. And of course, that's when our skin repairs itself, too—it's not called "beauty sleep" for nothing!

How to Make a "Clean Sleep"

One of my favorite expressions about this rule is "sleep hygiene." I love the idea that there is a systematic, pristine approach to bedtime, just like there is to washing your hands or brushing your teeth. And while I'm not saying I don't push it sometimes (I do fall asleep with my makeup on from time to time), I do try to follow these basic "hygiene" rules, which, sleep specialists have shown time and again, make it easier to fall asleep, stay asleep, and get the best quality sleep you possibly can.

• Banish all your electronics from the bedroom. Finding it a struggle to give up that phone? Allow yourself to check it before bedtime, then carefully put it to bed, too—away from your bedroom. I know it sounds silly, but some people think it actually helps to say "Goodnight, phone! See you in the morning!"

• Try to go to bed at the same time each evening and to get up about the same time in the morning—even on weekends and, yes, even on vacations. As nice as it feels to sleep in sometimes, it only makes it more difficult to maintain your bedtime discipline.

• Get moving! Exercise and activity during the day mean that when you fall asleep, you'll sleep more soundly, getting the high-quality rest you deserve.

• Get outdoors whenever you can. Regular exposure to the sun or bright lights, especially in the late afternoon, keeps your circadian rhythms in tune.

• Keep the temperature in your bedroom comfortable and consider wearing socks to bed if your feet get cold.

• Practice your eight-count breathing. Making mindfulness meditation part of your bedtime ritual will help you relax and make the transition from busy brain to sleepy head almost effortless.

• Pamper yourself. Maybe it's a cup of herbal tea, a rich hand cream, a spritz of fragrance on your pillow—a kind, gentle gesture that will help you remember you're about to enter your dreams. That's the ultimate "me" space!

Keri's Eight Favorite *Sweet-Dreams Foods*

Unfortunately, there's no food that works as a sleeping pill. For years, people believed turkey was a sleep-inducer because of the tryptophan it contains. Alas, researchers now know that there's no way a person could eat enough turkey to get such a result; instead, it's probably the way we overdo it with carbs on Thanksgiving that sends so many of us to the couch for a nap. That said, there are a number foods I'd like you to eat—and they're all included in the New You and Improved Diet plan. They won't knock you out like an Ambien, but they will soothe the stress and inflammation in the body, boost your cognitive function, and support healthy blood pressure. Combined, these things mean that when you do slip between the sheets at night, you'll drift off deep into dreamland!

APRICOTS Full of vitamin C and beta-carotene, apricots are one of the prettiest fruits ever, and I love their tangy-tart flavor. (Apricots have plenty of designer offspring, too, many crossed with plums—you'll find them with catchy names like Aprium, Plumcot, and Pluot.) Their connection to sleep? Stress resilience. Vitamin C–rich foods have been shown to help your body recover faster from stress, and fewer jangled nerves means mellower evenings. I like dried apricots, too—just be mindful of their higher calorie count and don't eat more than six halves per serving.

ASPARAGUS These delicate stalks are high in folate, which is essential for a healthy cardiovascular system and has a proven effect against anxiety. I like it fresh, but I always keep a few boxes of frozen asparagus tips on hand for nights when I run low on produce. Sautée them with some sliced almonds and a little cayenne for a fast and unexpected dish.

BANANA This sweet, creamy, and comforting tropical fruit is a good dietary source of melatonin, a hormone that aids sleep. Cranked out by our pineal gland, melatonin is secreted at night and helps regulate our body's natural rhythms. Since the amount we create drops sharply in the presence of either artificial or natural light, numerous studies have linked that decrease in nocturnal melatonin production to an increased risk of developing cancer. Bananas also have tryptophan (which we need to make

Best time of day to
Sleep

Just about anytime, as long as it's the same time every night. Sleep experts say that our bodies crave routines, and thanks to our circadian rhythms, our bodies are quite consistent. But, experts suggest, instead of thinking about when you feel like going to bed, you should focus on what time you need to get up and then back the schedule up by 8½ hours. That's because most people need 8 hours of sleep, and typically take 30 minutes to get ready for bed and fall asleep.

serotonin), as well as potassium, which helps normalize heartbeat. Some clients worry that bananas are fattening and shrink from my banana suggestion as if I'd told them to eat a hot fudge sundae before bedtime. At roughly 105 calories each and with all that nutrition, the humble banana is not to blame for America's obesity problem! But it is filling, and you don't have to eat the whole thing—just half at bedtime can make you feel full and sleepy. Then eat the other half with your breakfast the next day.

CHAMOMILE TEA Made from a tiny European flower that's in the daisy family, this tea, with its soothing mild flavor, is an age-old remedy for easing yourself to sleep. While there's not much clinical research to back this up yet, I've heard some health experts insist that chamomile tea can be more effective than sleeping pills, particularly if you get used to drinking it night after night! I like to brew myself a nice big mug before bedtime and sip it as I go through the last hour or so of my day.

CHICKPEAS These lovely legumes, whether smooshed into my beloved hummus, simmered in soups, or tossed into a salad, contain plenty of folate. Canned varieties are fine, but don't let the cooking time keep you from using the dried ones—use a quick-boil method and skip the whole overnight-soaking process.

NUTMEG While the smell might say something as simple as apple pie, researchers have shown that nutmeg improves blood pressure and cholesterol levels and also have found it to be effective against bacteria such as *E. coli*. And it's earned a reputation as a home remedy for anxiety, menstrual cramps, and even bad breath. Try a pinch in a glass of warm skim milk and watch how well you sleep.

POPCORN It's filling, and all that fiber makes it a great snack for someone trying to lose weight. It's also a significant source of antioxidants, with surprisingly large amounts of polyphenols. A 3-cup serving of popcorn, or about 100 calories, packs a powerful punch of fiber and stress-fighting serotonin, which can aid in a good night's sleep.

TART CHERRIES Considered a symbol of immortality in ancient China, these fruits are loaded with anthocyanins, an important type of antioxidant that lowers inflammation as well as cholesterol and triglyceride levels. But they're sleeping beauties, too—cherries are a source of melatonin, a hormone that aids sleep.

What Happens When You Don't Get Enough Sleep

You don't need me to tell you that you don't feel or perform your best when you're pooped. (And if you're like me, you don't look very good, either—I hate when I have bags under my eyes!) But plenty of other problems can arise from not getting enough sleep, besides the weight gain we've already discussed. They include:

YOU HAVE A GREATER RISK OF HIGH BLOOD PRESSURE

People with a poor quality of sleep are significantly more likely to develop blood pressure problems, reports the American Heart Association.

THE NEW YOU! Not only is this diet one of the most heart-healthy you'll ever meet, but it's also calming. Many of the foods on the plan have been specifically chosen because they ease inflammation, which is associated with many cardiovascular problems.

YOUR MEMORY GETS SCRAMBLED

Slow-wave sleep is important to memory processing, which is why we feel so scatterbrained and forgetful when we aren't sleeping well—it's because we really are forgetful! Turns out our brains can't consolidate new memories efficiently without enough solid z's.

THE NEW YOU! Certainly, I'm happy that the foods on the plan encourage good sleep habits. But so do all the other rules: Deep breathing and meditation have been shown to improve focus, for example, as has exercise. Remember, each of these rules support the others.

EVERYTHING HURTS MORE

Sleep experts at Johns Hopkins University in Baltimore studied a group of healthy young women and found that both too little sleep and frequently disrupted sleep made the women more susceptible to pain.

THE NEW YOU! Pampering yourself, developing the best exercise routine for your body, and learning to relax are all ways to baby yourself while you're losing weight.

Rule No. 8

Clean Out
Your Closet

Simplicity is the ultimate sophistication.
—LEONARDO DAVINCI

N ow that we've spent the last seven chapters focusing on the many things that are entirely under your control— what you eat and drink, how you exercise, sleep, and relax—it's time to take that New You thinking one step further, and it all starts with cleaning out your closet.

Of course, this is really all about improving the environment around you, though it doesn't quite seem fair to ask someone who is struggling to get a better grip on eating well, along with dealing with stress, exercising, and sleeping better, to fix global warming. Believe me, I want you to think about the whole planet. The more of us who are trying to help out Mother Nature, the better. And there are some big-picture environmental issues I hope we'll all spend more time thinking about. But I use the word *environment* in a much smaller sense, too. Sure, you're affected by what's happening in the world's oceans. But what's happening in your closet (and under your bathroom sink) is just as important.

How much clutter is on your nightstand? How much chaos is on your desk? How many different noises are bothering you right now, from your beeping BlackBerry to the TV in the other room or your neighbor's yapping dog? All of these things don't just affect how you feel (making you cranky or distracted without your really noticing). They can also have a major impact on your health and on how well you're able to follow the New You and Improved Diet.

Safeguard Your Home

I like to tell people to start very small when addressing this issue, and with the place they spend the most time: home, sweet home. To me, my home really is my castle. Once I'm home for the night—usually that means being barreled over by my kids, Maizy and Rex, the minute I walk in the door—I change into off-duty Keri, and I'm at my very happiest. Whether I'm playing with the kids, puttering around my kitchen, or just collapsing into my favorite spot on the couch (aaah!), I love that feeling of 100 percent safety, 100 percent relaxation, 100 percent . . . *me*.

But people's home (and office) environments can also be very stressful. And believe it or not, simple clutter is a big factor: One recent Australian study found that 88 percent of people think they have too much clutter at home, and for 40 percent of them, it causes genuine stress and anxiety. Spending an hour to reorganize your closet will save you plenty of stress—and time—in the long run. Getting dressed shouldn't be an act of aggravation; it should be easy. Taking things you haven't worn in ages to a charity will free up space. And even the simplest concepts can help: Divvying up your closet between weekend and work clothes, separating clothing by season, and even buying a shoe bag can all cut down on frantic rummaging around in the mornings.

Clean Out Your Closet:
HOW IT CONNECTS

Taking control of the environment all around you—from your closet to the planet—reinforces every rule, but it's especially critical to eating well (Rule No. 1), managing stress (Rule No. 2), and making sure you're hydrated (Rule No. 3). These simple steps toward controlling clutter and eliminating dangerous chemicals will make it easier for you to be healthy, calm, and in control.

As you begin the New You and Improved Diet, don't feel like you have to be too ambitious in tackling anything big, but here's a trick that always works for me: Walk through the house with a laundry basket and just start tossing clutter into it—magazines you've been meaning to read, bottles of nail polish you've been meaning to organize, whatever. Stick it in a closet. I promise, when you're in the mood to tackle it, it will all still be there. And meanwhile, you'll be able to relax a little because you've simplified your space.

From there, have a quick look around another place you spend a lot of time: your office. Take a half hour to clean everything off your desk, including your computer. Before you put anything back, ask yourself if you really need it and if it's arranged in the way that's most comfortable for you. Are the things you use the most the closest to you? Can you reach everything you need? Is your desk organized in a way that makes you feel capable, or does it make you feel jittery and anxious? Is there something pretty you can add—a potted plant, a memento from a favorite trip?

Next, tackle your car. Spend 5 minutes sitting and thinking about what would make your drive time less stressful and a better experience for you. What would make the space more organized and helpful? An easy first step is to take out the unnecessary things—the extra shoes, the coffee cups, the broken ice scrapers. After you start taking junk out, you can start to think about what you might bring in. I know people who keep an extra bag of makeup in the console so they can apply it while sitting quietly in the parking lot between the gym and work. Others stash a pair of sneakers in the trunk so they can always be ready for a walk. Maybe stocking a handful of nuts in resealable plastic bags in the glove compartment would be a lifesaver the next time you get stuck in traffic. An aromatherapy dispenser that slips into the cigarette lighter might be soothing. The point is, your car is just as much a part of your life as any other place, so why not give it a makeover that will add to your sense of control?

CLEAN UP THE AIR THAT YOU BREATHE

Carbon dioxide, carbon monoxide, ozone—air pollutants are a big problem that affects the health of each and every one of us, as well as the planet. And while it may seem like our individual actions won't have

Best time of day to **Exercise Outdoors:**
Early or Late

Running is one of the biggest treats in my life, and not just for the exercise—it's also my therapy and a fun way to explore the world. Whether I'm at home in New York City or traveling, an early-morning run makes me feel like a world-class adventurer.

But I hate the idea that the air I'm breathing in might be hurting me more than the exercise is helping me. And I think it's totally unfair that the risks of this are the highest in summer, which is when most of us want to go outside and play!

Summer's combination of higher temperatures and fewer breezes mean the air stagnates, especially ozone, an invisible gas created when sunlight triggers a chemical reaction between oxygen-containing molecules and pollution from cars, power plants, factories, and other sources. So, on bad air days, try to schedule your outdoor exercise and activity for either late in the evening or early in the morning. Ozone levels generally reach their highest levels between midafternoon and early evening.

Clean Your Air,
Brighten Your Mood

Even when you think you've taken as many steps as possible to breathe clean air in your home or office, there are still traces of chemicals hanging around. Mother Nature uses plants to clean up the mess, and you should, too. NASA has researched the effect common houseplants have on indoor air pollutants and says the following plants do the best job of minimizing such toxins as formaldehyde, benzene, and carbon monoxide. And for those of us with not-the-greenest thumbs, the good news is they are also fairly easy to grow:

Bamboo palm
Chinese evergreen
English ivy
Gerbera daisy
Janet Craig dracaena
Marginata dracaena

Mass cane/Corn plant
Mother-in-law's tongue
Peace lily
Pot mum
Warneckii dracaena

much of an impact on our city's (or global) air quality, it's important that we be as conscientious as possible in the ways we vote, shop, and live.

We can have a big impact on the air we breathe inside our own home. Believe it or not, many experts think the air we breathe at home is dirtier than what we breathe outdoors, even in cities. Here are two ways the Environmental Protection Agency suggests we can clean up:

OPEN THE WINDOWS On one hand, we've all been encouraged to keep our homes tight and snug, as a way to improve energy efficiency and lower heating and cooling bills. And that's great, because when we use less fuel, we help the world's atmosphere. But on the other hand, it can create ventilation problems. Use the kitchen and bathroom fans frequently, and every so often, throw your windows open for 15 minutes or so to let the bad air out and the good air in. (Obviously, this isn't a good strategy if you live in a very polluted area, such as near a freeway. A recent study found that people who lived within 328 feet of a freeway were twice as likely to develop hardening of the arteries as those who lived farther away.)

LOOK FOR LOW-FUME PRODUCTS Volatile organic compounds (VOCs) are in almost every product in our homes, with paint, carpets, and furniture being the most problematic. Over a 6-month period, most of these fumes and gases dissipate, but some linger for years. Studies have even found traces of them in breast milk. Shop for low-VOC products, and be especially attentive to ventilation when you redecorate or renovate.

FRESHEN UP THE FRIDGE

Making the inside of your refrigerator look welcoming, organized—even pretty!—will set you up for success on the plan. It's the difference between opening the door after a long day and saying, "Wow, imagine the healthy possibilities!" and well, "Blechhh."

OUT WITH THE OLD. Most people have the doors of their fridge lined with past-the-sell-by-date condiments, sticky jars of relish or jelly, and crusty little packages of leftovers. Throw out anything you haven't used recently and anything that you think might tempt you to make a poor choice. Do you really need eight kinds of fatty salad dressing?

SPOTLIGHT THE NEW. Rearrange your shelves so the first thing you'll look at are the healthiest items. I like to keep a glass carafe of water, maybe with cucumber or lemon slices, prepped on the main shelf, as well as almond milk for my coffee. On the lower shelves, I have tubs of yogurt and cottage cheese readily visible. And I'm careful to keep the crisper drawers current, so when I see my turnip greens looking too wilty, a limp cucumber, or a puckered yellow pepper, I know it's time to use them up, maybe in a soup or a stir-fry.

SHOW OFF YOUR PREP PROWESS. On weekends, I try to get ready for the week ahead and make sure to stack that prep work up in neat, organized glass containers. For me, that includes prechopping things like peppers, celery, and carrots, so I can toss them into salads and recipes as needed. But it also usually means doubling up a soup, grilling chicken, or boiling eggs, so I always have an easy base to a meal. (If I'm really ambitious, I'll make enough to freeze, too, so I always have something to fill the fridge with, even if I haven't had a chance to go shopping.)

My Favorite Cleaning Products

These are a few brands that I love: Seventh Generation, Method, and Sun and Earth. But if you prefer to make your own, try these suggestions.

Lemon. I always have lemons at home. I have a stash of sliced or wedged lemons in my refrigerator at all times to toss into a glass of water or to squeeze on my salad or fish. There is no denying that they are a staple in my world, and I love lemon for liver support, vitamin C burst, and fresh scent. In my home, I use lemons to clean, and I love this product <https://opensky.com/keriglassman/product/full-circle-home--diy-natural-home-cleaning-kit-kg> to make my own cleaning solution. I squeeze a lemon into a spray bottle and wipe down my countertops. It works beautifully to remove grease without chemicals. It can also be used as a bleaching agent on clothing, so if I accidentally have a spill at a restaurant, I ask for a slice of lemon to treat a potential stain.

White vinegar. I use white vinegar in cucumber and tomato salads (instead of mayonnaise), and I love the role of all vinegars in my health and wellness. For no calories but tons of flavor, vinegar aids the digestive system; it contains potassium, magnesium, calcium, pectin, and acetic acid. It improves the absorption and utilization of several essential nutrients. When I am in doubt about how to clean something, white vinegar is my usual go-to. I use it mixed with a little water (and sometimes a bit of castile soap) on my floors, windows, and shower doors and in toilets and drains. I'm always thrilled when I smell vinegar because I know my home is clean.

Baking soda. An obvious choice as a cleaning product, baking soda is not just used to make your dough rise. Most of us have this baking staple all over our homes to absorb odors. I keep a box in the pantry, one in the fridge, one in the freezer, and one in the closet with my kids' sports equipment. While I often don't change the boxes often enough (change every 30 days!), I am comforted to know they are there. There is not much nutritional benefit to baking soda. Still, baking soda is a cleaning powerhouse and can be mixed with a little water to form a paste and clean grout between bathroom tiles, sterling silver, and stains on china and ceramics. Also, there is nothing better at removing red wine. Simply pour the baking soda over the stain (as soon as you can), let it dry, and all of the wine will transfer to the baking soda. Vacuum it up and no one will be the wiser!

Olive oil. A prince among oils, olive oil contains those wonderful monounsaturated fatty acids that are cardio-protective; it can improve cholesterol profiles when used in the place of other fats and provides delicious satiety. It is also used in my beauty routine as a moisturizer for my hair, nails, and skin and in my home care routine as a wood polish! Used to return shine to otherwise dull or untreated wood, simply combine 3 parts olive oil to 1 part vinegar or lemon juice.

TURN DOWN THE SOUND

We live in a noisy world, and a lot of it is self-inflicted. (I know, I know. I'm guilty of occasionally cranking up my earphones too loud, too.) It goes without saying that it's bad for our hearing. And most of us are aware, at least occasionally, that too much sound from too many different sources makes us distracted and less efficient. Environmental noise, even when we aren't conscious of it, affects our sleep cycle. It interferes with our memory and may make us more aggressive. It's also associated with cardiovascular disease, high blood pressure, and certain psychiatric disorders.

Of course, you can't do much about the planes, trains, and cars in the world around you. But you can control your buffer zones. In your yard, for example, carefully planted trees can muffle noise, and water fountains can add white noise to soften sounds. Within your home, start with simple changes. Are TVs or radios often on in multiple rooms? Can you turn the volume down on phone ringers? If traffic or neighbors are noisy, look into sound drapes and white noise machines. There are even alarm clocks that can wake you up gradually, using your favorite sounds—gentle waves, singing birds, or chirping frogs. Switch the ringtone on your phone to something soothing, like chimes or chirps.

FIND YOUR DARK SIDE

While everyone knows that sunshine improves our mood, it's easy to forget we need the reverse, too. Ever since Edison invented the lightbulb, sitting in the dark has been more or less optional. But there's a downside, and researchers now know that constant light can disrupt our circadian rhythms, with some pretty extreme consequences. Scientists have even established a link between women working night shifts and breast cancer. Some researchers speculate that it might have to do with melatonin, the hormone we talked about in Rule No. 7. Melatonin is secreted at night and is important in regulating our body's natural rhythms. Since the amount we create drops sharply in the presence of either artificial or natural light, numerous studies have linked that decrease in nocturnal melatonin production to an increased risk of developing cancer.

Take 5 minutes to see how you can make your bedroom darker, either by fully closing the drapes (it's worth buying new ones that block out more light) or by removing the many gadgets that cast a light in the room—TVs, DVRs, cellphone chargers, you name it. Too draconian? I have clients who just cover up the displays by leaning a book over them at night, and that includes covering their alarm clock. It works!

Buy the Cleanest Food Possible

People in my line of work spend a lot of time studying the basic components of food and looking at data about what certain chemicals and additives might do, in terms of the nutritional value of a food as well as the risks they might pose. And of course, we all know that the more real a food is, the better.

So if I ruled the world, we would all eat nothing but the finest organic produce, preferably in season. It would come from local sources, so that it wouldn't have to be shipped thousands of miles by trucks spewing exhaust into the air. We'd eat lots of whole-grain products, like deliciously crusty and chewy artisanal breads, baked by people we know in our hometowns. We'd get our yogurt, cheese, and milk products from friendly nearby farms. Even our meat would be local, and we could guarantee that each cow, pig, and chicken had grazed on plenty of good healthy stuff, frolicked in the sunshine, and been butchered following the highest standards. (I know, I sound like I just fell out of an episode of *Portlandia,* don't I?)

But very few of us can live like that. Organic produce, while it has been shown to be somewhat more nutritious for people and far better for the environment, is still a bit pricier than conventionally grown produce. (I am happy to report that's changing all the time, as more and more farmers jump on the organic bandwagon and as farmers' markets become available to more and more people.)

The price difference is still quite pronounced in proteins, and as much as I love grass-fed beef and wild-caught salmon, I'm keenly aware that not everyone can or chooses to pay that much for food all the time.

Whatever you do, don't go nuts about this. You can't be all or nothing, and if you try to make the best decision about everything, you'll quickly find yourself paralyzed by the overwhelming amount of information (much of it conflicting). Don't feel like you're doing something bad if you're committed to a certain kind of cleaner—just try to make a greener choice in another area. Buy wild salmon to eat at home, for example, but don't give yourself a hard time for ordering farmed salmon in a restaurant.

I'm also aware that not every decision should be based purely on nutrition. Some experts might argue that it's better for the planet in the

Cutting Down on Plastics

Like many people, I'm concerned about a chemical called BPA that's in many plastics, and I try to avoid buying products that include it. There are concerns that this chemical, which mimics estrogen, can harm children and fetuses, and there is growing evidence that it's also connected to rising obesity and diabetes rates.

But an important 2011 study, which tested 450 plastic products ranging from sippy cups to can linings to plastic wraps, found that other chemicals, even in BPA-free products, released the same estrogen-like chemicals. While the study, published in *Environmental Health Perspectives*, didn't look for health risks but rather traces of these chemicals, it's enough to make experts wary of many more plastics. Since then, I've been trying to use glass containers whenever possible, and I suggest you do the same.

Yes, there are practical reasons why I still use plastic occasionally—for example, glass is heavy and can break. When I do use plastic, I use brands made from high-density polyethylene (HDPE, or plastic #2), low-density polyethylene (LDPE, or plastic #4), and polypropylene (PP, or plastic #5), which are considered the safest, including Tupperware, Glad, Hefty, Ziploc, and Saran. (These have all been tested by the Green Guide, which is a good resource for environmental and health information. Find it at environment.nationalgeographic.com/environment/green-guide).

long run if you eat locally grown produce that isn't organic, meaning it's been raised with fertilizers and pesticides, rather than organic produce that's been shipped in from, let's say, China. (The argument is that we need to make some tradeoffs that give the environment priority over our personal health concerns.) In fact, new research from Mintel, a company that tracks how consumers spend their food money, reports that 52 percent of American shoppers now think that buying local produce matters more than buying organic. That's a big shift from several years ago.

And even though I make most of my own choices based on the quality of the food, I try not to argue with people about their decisions. Food issues are complex, and everyone's got to find the balance between ethical and practical that works for them.

That said, chemicals cause problems. Take the apple, which I think of as one of Mother Nature's best ideas *ever*. Recently, the US Department of Agriculture found residues of pesticides in a staggering 98 percent of the apples it tested, by far the highest rate of any type of produce. While in almost every case the USDA ruled that the amount of the harmful chemicals was within its "safe" levels, I don't want to eat them! The USDA's findings even prompted the Environmental Working Group, an influential watchdog organization, to put conventionally grown apples on its "Dirty Dozen" list. (Check out its "Dirty Dozen," "Clean 15," and other really useful lists at ewg.org.)

The truth is, with so many scientists studying the food chain from so many different angles, new information comes to light all the time. So it's up to all of us to stay abreast of changes. I like to shop at places like Whole Foods Market, Trader Joe's, and my local health food stores because I'm more likely to find someone willing to explain the differences between, let's say, two types of canned tuna. And farmers' markets are great because you can often get insight from the people who've grown the food, from recipes to advice about freezing to information about organic practices.

FOR BEEF, TREAT YOURSELF TO GRASS-FED, AT LEAST SOMETIMES.
I love grass-fed beef. It's not just because it's lower in calories, and has

more omega-3 fats and such antioxidants as vitamins A and E and perhaps seven times as much beta-carotene. I think it tastes much, much better, too. But it also costs a typical beef eater about $300 more a year, which isn't chicken feed. I think it's one thing that's worth the splurge!

FOR SALMON, GO WITH WILD-CAUGHT FRESH FOR SPECIAL OCCASIONS. Again, in my perfect world, everyone would eat wild-caught salmon three times a week. But candidly, if that happened, we'd all be in trouble—there just aren't enough of these wonderful fish in the oceans to feed us all. That means we're going to have to eat farmed fish, at least some of the time. This does worry me, since some studies have shown that farmed salmon are more likely to contain polychlorinated biphenyls (PCBs), a pollutant linked to cancer. (And honestly, how good can a registered dietitian feel about recommending salmon for heart health and a calmer mood while knowing it may increase your cancer risk?)

But with wild-caught salmon, there's no guarantee against contamination and pollutants, either. (Hey, it's not like the fish tell us where they've been swimming the last few years!) And one important study found that wild-caught salmon in the Pacific Northwest (the major supplier of wild-caught salmon for most of the United States) contain higher rates of mercury than farmed.

So, my advice is to splurge on the wild-caught stuff, feel okay about eating the farm-raised, if that's the only option, and stay tuned—we are learning more about sustainability every day. And by the way, salmon isn't the only fish in town. Go to seafoodwatch.org to stay on top of the healthiest and most sustainable options.

CONTINUE TO MONITOR YOUR PACKAGED FOOD PURCHASES. Over the years, packaged foods, which are generally highly processed and heavy on chemical preservatives and artificial coloring, have been losing favor with more demanding consumers. And many experts believe there is a link between the chemicals used in many packaged foods and the obesity epidemic: The strongest evidence focuses on preservatives,

MSG, and high-fructose corn syrup. And bisphenol A (BPA), present in canned foods, has been identified as a potential obesogen.

I'm happy to report that the concern has made its way from food gurus to mainstream American households. In the past decade, sales of fresh foods have skyrocketed, while sales of processed foods have actually fallen. That's not to say all processed food is bad. As a busy mom, I know there are some days when the world just can't go around without using some of these quick and easy solutions. But even among packaged foods, you can make choices that involve fewer chemicals and more whole foods. (See my portion guide for some of my favorite brands on page 245.)

Reevaluate Your Water

One of the things that has always made Americans so healthy, compared with populations in other parts of the world, is our great water supply—in so many places, the plumbing and the water availability we take for granted are considered a luxury. But our water supply system is not perfect, and increasingly, everyone from public health experts to infrastructure engineers is becoming worried about what's in our H_2O.

More than 20 percent of the country's water-treatment plants, providing water to 49 million people, have violated water-safety laws, piping water that contains things like arsenic, radioactive traces of uranium, and even raw sewage into people's homes.

And even those of us who live in areas with good water can have bacteria, lead, copper, or traces from plastics leach into water from home plumbing. Scientists estimate that 7 million Americans are sickened by contaminated tap water every year, and that nearly 40 percent of our rivers fail to meet current clean water standards.

Unfortunately, bottled water isn't a good answer. For one thing,

"Keri, what about the chemicals in sunscreen?"

I adore being outside, and an early-morning run when the world is waking up is my idea of sun-drenched bliss. I've always thought it was incredibly amazing that our bodies are smart enough to convert sunshine—a nonfood—into vitamin D, an essential nutrient.

But the UV rays in sunshine are an environmental hazard, too, and a major source of oxidative damage. I know you don't need me to tell you to wear sunscreen, and it's great the way more and more products now contain adequate SPF.

I look for sunscreens that use zinc oxide (and are fragrance and paraben-free), rather than benzophenone-3 (BP-3), which has been linked to some disturbing problems in animal studies.

there's no guarantee that it's any cleaner. A report from the Environmental Working Group found that only 3 of the 173 bottled waters surveyed (and just one of the top US brands) tell customers the source of the water and how it's been treated.

And while drinking eight glasses of tap water a day will cost you about 49 cents per year, reports the *New York Times,* drinking that same amount of bottled water will cost about $1,400 per year. In 2007, Americans consumed more than 50 billion single-serve bottles of water. Yes, I'm thrilled that that means soda consumption is declining. But it also means that between 30 million and 40 million single-serve bottles went into landfills each year.

The best fix? A home water filter—either a water pitcher filter you use on your countertop or the type you install on your faucet. Prices vary, as does the complexity. Carve out a Saturday afternoon in the next few weeks to do some reading on your local water quality, and come up with a plan of filtration that might work for you. Again, don't go nuts here, because some conversations about filtration get so complex it can be overwhelming, and I don't want you to give yourself nightmares about things like arsenic and cryptosporidium! But clean water is important, so educating yourself is a good first step.

Keri's Eight Favorite
Antioxidant Foods

When it comes to warding off the destructive environmental forces we all run into—even in the most pristine of environments—I'm happy to report that the antioxidant-rich foods I'm such a fan of are among the most healthful allies we've got. For the New You and Improved Diet, I've chosen foods so high on the ORAC scale of antioxidant powers that they're practically superheroes.

Don't get me wrong. Almost all plant-based foods contain some type of antioxidant capabilities, meaning they possess chemicals and properties that can help corral damaging free radicals, which cause disease and aging. In fact, though the study of these antioxidants is still in its infancy, relatively speaking, we know there are likely hundreds of thousands of them, even if researchers haven't yet isolated, named, or tested for them. Some that we do know, right now, are positively off the ORAC charts. By now, if you're following the plan, I've already vaulted you into the elite leagues of antioxidant consumption. But here are eight more of my high-ORAC favorites that may have escaped your attention so far. Please eat them often!

AMARANTH The Aztecs loved this grain, which tastes sweet and kind of nutty and is a good source of iron, magnesium, and zinc. I add the seeds to soups and stews, or cook it in a little sesame oil and serve it in place of rice. Even the leaves are edible—they taste like spinach. I like to have it as a hot cereal sometimes; it takes about 25 minutes but is worth the wait!

BLACK RICE BRAN This variety of rice may be a novelty here, but it's a staple food for one-third of the world's population. Available at stores like Whole Foods Market, the bran—or outer coating of the rice grain— is loaded with anthocyanins, as many as are in blueberries. These phytochemicals, found in many purple and reddish foods, are linked to a decreased risk of heart disease and cancer and improvements in memory.

Try black rice bran the next time you make rice as a side dish, or use it in a vegetable-filled risotto.

CANTALOUPE Refreshing and sweet, this melon is also a nutrient gold mine: A single serving of cantaloupe provides you with more than your recommended dietary allowance of vitamin A. We all know that types of vitamin A work wonders when applied directly to the skin—that's why we're buying up all those retinol products! But we need to eat foods rich in vitamin A to keep our skin smooth and our eyesight sharp, and it's a good buffer against damaging free radicals. Cantaloupe isn't just for breakfast—chunk one up and serve it with raspberries and almonds for dessert.

EGGPLANT Not only does this vegetable—a staple in Italian foods—have high levels of chlorogenic acid, one of the most powerful antioxidants found in plants; it also has 13 other phenolic acids. And here's the kind of research factoid that floors me: While analyzing some wild eggplants, researchers found several phenolic compounds that had never before been isolated. There's potentially a whole new antioxidant frontier, right there in Eggplantville! Grill it, sliced lengthwise, with a little olive oil, sea salt, and rosemary—it's easy and delicious!

PECANS All nuts tend to be rich in vitamin E, a powerful antioxidant, as well as a good source of protein and heart-healthy fats. (Plus they're so satisfying that working them into your diet as, let's say, a midmorning or midafternoon snack ensures you won't show up at your next meal too hungry to think.) Pecans have the highest antioxidant power and have been shown to reduce lipid oxidation—a critical measure of heart health—by 7.4 percent. They also contain plant sterols, which lower cholesterol. Even the Food and Drug Administration agrees, and suggests that eating 1½ ounces of nuts, such as pecans, each day lowers the risk of heart disease. Eight halves contain 2,500 ORAC points, and because pecans are a little sweeter, they can cure a candy craving.

PISTACHIOS For many people, these nuts are a great diet tool, since it takes time to pop the little green guys out of their shells, meaning you

Ingredients to Avoid

Artificial sweeteners
  (sucralose, acesulfame
  potassium, Saccharin,
  aspartame)
Butylated hydroxyanisole
  (BHA) and butylated
  hydroxytoluene (BHT)

Artificial food colorings
High-fructose corn syrup
Monosodium glutamate
  (MSG)
Partially hydrogenated oils
Sodium nitrate and nitrite
Soy protein isolate

For a more complete list and updated information, check out my Web site at www.nutritiouslife.com.

eat them more slowly. Like pecans, pistachios are packed with plant sterols, which researchers believe might lower the risk of heart disease and which have been shown to reduce the risk of lung and other cancers. Eighteen pistachios have 1,000 ORAC points. They're a perfect party food: I'm always amazed that a bowl of pistachios draws almost as big a crowd as a bowl of my guacamole!

RED BEANS I've already raved about black beans and chickpeas, but don't overlook red beans, both the smalls ones and the larger kidney beans. Both have well over 13,000 ORAC points per serving, and they make a great addition to just about any salad, stir-fry, soup, or stew.

RUSSET POTATOES Yep, here I am, a nutritionist, giving my blessing to potatoes! In the last decade of carb bashing, the poor spud has gotten a bad rap. Of course, when we turn them into french fries or mash them with way too much butter, they're not a good choice. But a whole baked russet potato provides 4,600 ORAC points and is a great source of vitamin C, which is so helpful in combating free radicals, and vitamin B_6 and potassium, which are good for your heart. Look for a medium-size potato (which is likely to have about 190 calories, making it a good "base" for your meal). I like mine topped with plenty of salsa and a small portion of reduced-fat Monterey Jack cheese.

What Happens When Your World Is Too Polluted

Keeping up with the tsunami of new information about the many ways we've put our environment in peril can be exhausting. Sometimes I feel like I spend my days advocating for one health change, only to get it shot down by new information. "Eat more fish oil. But wait, look out for the mercury!" "Consume more healthy antioxidants from produce! Hold on, those cranberries may deliver a terrifying pesticide-per-serving risk!" But just because much of the emerging data is still unclear (and often controversial) doesn't mean there isn't plenty of solid science we can act on, starting right now. We know, for example, that pollution means:

WE BREATHE BADLY AND CANCER RATES RISE

Air pollution is not only linked to asthma and respiratory distress; it's also related to 3 percent of all American deaths. And around the world, all forms of pollution are connected to 40 percent of deaths, many of them due to waterborne diseases.

THE NEW YOU! Antioxidants are proven protectors against the oxidative damages causes by everything from the sun to air pollution to harmful chemicals. It's not a bulletproof shield, of course. Nothing can protect us fully from these assaults. But dietary antioxidants—the kind you'll be eating all day long on the plan—have been proved to help.

CLUTTER MAKES US CRAZY

When our environment gets too cluttered and complicated, it makes it hard for us to focus, and we get distracted without realizing it. Researchers at the Princeton University Neuroscience Institute have studied the way too many things crowding and competing for our visual attention can simply slow down our ability to process *anything*. (Of course, you didn't exactly need Ivy League brain scientists to tell you that trying to find your car keys on a cluttered kitchen counter is a lot more aggravating than hanging them on a hook by the door each time, did you?)

THE NEW YOU! I've loaded the plan with foods that have lots of nutrients proven to support what researchers call "cognitive function" and what I call the ability to find my keys! Those include choices naturally rich in vitamin E, fatty acids found in fish, vitamin B_{12}, and folate.

THE ATMOSPHERE THINS AND WE BECOME MORE VULNERABLE

With less ozone in the air to protect us from the sun's UVB rays, the Environmental Protection Agency says we increase our risks of sunburn, skin cancer, and cataracts. These UVB rays also mess with phytoplankton in the oceans, disrupting the food chain.

THE NEW YOU! Again, focusing on antioxidants, both in skin care products and in our diets, can minimize those risks.

PART 2

the

NEW
YOU
(and improved!)
DIET
PLAN

Whether you are already an accomplished cook or the kind of person who spends as little time in the kitchen as possible, I hope you'll spend some time leafing through these recipes, even before you head out to the grocery store or start dicing red peppers. That's because I'm convinced a handful will "speak" to you, right off the bat, and I want you to listen carefully. Part of the way people discover the path toward a healthier pattern of eating is by tuning in to that voice—often, it is not only telling you what you like, but what you *need*. And in our food-crazy culture, it's too easy to learn to ignore those innate preferences that we all have. Why is it that some mornings, an egg burrito sounds like heaven, while on another, some combo of oats and peanut butter feels like the best idea ever? It's because your body is trying to get your attention, directing you toward the optimal foods for you, right now.

So start reading, listen up, and . . . enjoy!

The New You and Improved Diet Recipes

<hr/>

Whether it's a new twist on something you already love or a whole new type of food, I'm sure five or ten of these recipes will easily become favorites you'll savor for years.

But for now, be as open-minded as you can. In the early weeks of the plan, your taste buds will awaken to the power of these clean, real foods. You'll be dazzled by the impact of even the most basic ingredients, whether it's a dab of Dijon mustard, a quick blast of red pepper flakes, or the perfection of a spiced fig or a sweet potato wedge.

    Note: The recipes without a serving size are made to serve one.

Recipe Key

GF Gluten-free (*Note:* See asterisks throughout for additional information.)

VEG Vegetarian (*Note:* These are not vegan and some recipes include seafood.)

NC No cook/prep in advance (***Note:*** "Microwave" meals are considered no-cook.)

Be a locavore

Research a local food that's in season and work it into this week's meal plan.

Breakfast

Monday Morning Detox

`GF` `VEG` `NC`

½ Anjou pear, chopped
¾ cup low-fat or almond milk
2 teaspoons almond butter
¼ teaspoon minced ginger or ⅛ teaspoon ground
½ teaspoon matcha green tea powder
½ cup frozen raspberries

1. Blend all ingredients except the raspberries until smooth.

2. Add the raspberries to the blender and pulse until smooth. Pour into a tall glass and serve.

Be a cayenne cowgirl!
Experiment with this hot spice on at least one food today to speed weight loss. Some studies have shown it increases weight loss by up to 25 percent.

Easy Date-Nut Clusters

¼   cup hazelnuts

1½   cups old-fashioned rolled oats*

½   cup quinoa, rinsed and drained

3   tablespoons chia seeds

2   teaspoons ground cinnamon

¼   teaspoon ground cloves

¼   teaspoon ground nutmeg

¼   teaspoon sea salt

2   egg whites

¼   cup pure maple syrup or honey

¼   cup pitted and finely chopped Medjool dates (about 2)

1. Preheat the oven to 350°F. Line 2 baking sheets with parchment paper and place the hazelnuts in a single layer on top of one of them. Bake the nuts for 10 minutes, or until they're fragrant and lightly browned. Let cool completely.

Make a conscious decision

to shut down the kitchen as soon as you finish cleaning up the dinner dishes. Studies have shown that the darker it gets, the poorer our food choices are.

THE NEW YOU AND IMPROVED DIET RECIPES

2. Combine the oats, quinoa, chia seeds, cinnamon, cloves, nutmeg, and salt in a large bowl. Finely chop the hazelnuts and stir them into the mixture.

3. Whisk the egg whites in another bowl until foamy. Add them to the mixture along with the maple syrup, stirring to coat. Gently stir in the dates.

4. Scoop scant ¼ cupfuls of the mixture onto the parchment-lined baking sheets about 2 inches apart. Gently pat into 2" rounds. Bake in the center of the oven for 15 to 20 minutes, or until the edges are lightly browned, turning the baking sheets once halfway through.

5. Let the clusters cool completely on the baking sheets. Serve with 1 cup of fat-free milk. Store in an airtight container for up to 1 week.

Makes 6 servings (3 clusters per serving)

* Use oats labeled gluten-free.

Double up
Think of at least two recipes you can double, and stash half of each in the fridge or freezer.

Melon & Mint Medley

`GF` `VEG` `NC`

2   tablespoons 100% pomegranate juice
1   cup fat-free plain or Greek yogurt
½   cup cubed seedless watermelon
1   small kiwifruit, peeled and cut into ½" pieces
1   tablespoon finely chopped mint
1   teaspoon honey
8   pecan halves

1. Stir the pomegranate juice into the yogurt.

2. Toss the watermelon and kiwifruit with the mint and honey in a small bowl.

3. In a small bowl, layer one-quarter of the fruit mixture, then one-third of the yogurt mixture, and top with one-third of the pecans. Repeat the layers twice, finishing with remaining fruit mixture.

Clean out your pantry
Spend 5 minutes pulling out items that might tempt you, that you don't like, or that you will never use—and donate them to the local food pantry.

Better-Than-Cereal Bowl

⅓   cup hot cooked bulgur*
¼   cup unsweetened applesauce
¼   teaspoon ground cinnamon
¼–½ teaspoon pure almond extract
    (such as Frontier brand)
½   cup fresh dark sweet cherries, pitted and halved,
    or frozen, thawed
1   tablespoon chopped, dry-roasted, unsalted,
    or raw almonds

1. Combine the bulgur, applesauce, cinnamon, and almond extract in a small bowl.

2. Gently stir in the cherries and almonds and add additional cinnamon if desired.

3. Serve with 1 cup of fat-free or almond milk.

* Substitute hot cooked quinoa for the bulgur.

Your phone is your friend
If you can't write down your food,
track it here!

Caribbean Pineapple & Papaya Cup

2/3 cup part-skim ricotta cheese
2   tablespoons unsweetened shredded coconut
Dash ground nutmeg
1/2 cup diced pineapple
1/4 cup green grapes, halved, or 1 kiwifruit, chopped
1   tablespoon chopped dried papaya or dried mango
1   teaspoon lime juice

1. Combine the ricotta, coconut, and nutmeg in a small bowl.

2. Combine the pineapple, grapes, papaya, and lime juice in another small bowl.

3. In a tall glass, layer one-quarter of the fruit mixture, then one-third of the ricotta mixture. Repeat the layers twice, ending with the remaining fruit.

Simplify portion control
by stashing measuring cups and spoons in an easy-to-reach drawer or cupboard.

Peanut Butter Cup Oatmeal

`GF*` `VEG` `NC`

½ cup old-fashioned rolled oats*
¾ cup low-fat milk
2 teaspoons smooth peanut butter
2 teaspoons dark chocolate chips

1. Combine the oats and milk in a small bowl with a dash of salt. Microwave on high for 2 to 3 minutes, stirring halfway through and again after the oats are cooked through.

2. Stir the peanut butter into the oats mixture until well combined.

3. Top with dark chocolate chips.

* Use oats labeled gluten-free.

Downsize your china

Eating from smaller dishes—like dessert plates rather than dinner plates—is a proven way to aid weight loss. Studies have shown that those who switch from a 12-inch plate to a 10-inch plate consume 22 percent fewer calories.

Herbed Egg Burrito

GF

1   large omega-3-enriched egg

2   tablespoons fat-free milk

2   tablespoons shredded mozzarella or Cheddar cheese

1   tablespoon finely chopped fresh basil

¼   teaspoon dried oregano

⅛   teaspoon garlic powder

1   teaspoon cold-pressed olive oil

¼   cup chopped yellow onion

¼   cup chopped red bell pepper

1   cup baby spinach

2   slices (2 ounces) uncured, nitrate-free deli ham (such as Applegate Naturals), chopped

1   (12 ounce) brown rice tortilla (such as Food for Life brand)

Keep a deck of cards
on your kitchen counter—it's a great visual reminder of how big a typical protein serving should be.

1. Combine the egg, milk, cheese, basil, oregano, and garlic powder in a small bowl. Season with salt and freshly ground black pepper.

2. Heat the oil in a small nonstick skillet over medium heat.

3. Place the onion and pepper in the skillet and cook for 2 to 3 minutes, or until softened. Add the spinach and ham and cook for 1 to 2 minutes more, until the spinach is just wilted.

4. Add the egg mixture to the skillet and reduce the heat to medium-low. Cook for 2 to 3 more minutes, or until the egg is cooked through, stirring frequently to scramble. Remove the skillet from the heat.

5. Place the tortilla flat between 2 damp paper towels and microwave for 20 to 30 seconds, until heated throughout.

6. Place the egg mixture on one side of the tortilla, leaving a 1" border on all sides, and tuck the ends in before rolling it up.

Going out to eat?
Have your strategy ready, whether it's checking the menu ahead of time, splitting an entrée, asking for sauce or dressing on the side.

Spiced Fig & Ricotta Toast

VEG NC

⅓ cup low-fat ricotta cheese
½ teaspoon pure maple syrup or honey
¼ teaspoon ground cinnamon
⅛ teaspoon ground nutmeg
¼ teaspoon minced ginger or ⅛ teaspoon ground
1 tablespoon chopped walnuts
1 whole wheat english muffin, toasted
1 Black Mission fig, cut lengthwise into ¼"-thick slices,
   or 2 dried, halved

1. Combine the cheese, maple syrup, cinnamon, nutmeg, ginger, and walnuts in a small bowl.

2. Divide the mixture on top of the English muffin halves. Place the fig slices flat on top of the ricotta mixture and serve open-faced.

Canned food safari

Dare yourself to walk down the canned goods aisle and grab three new foods to try, such as a healthy soup, a new kind of bean, or sardines. Remember to look for BPA-free.

Nutritious Life Power Bars

2	cups old-fashioned rolled oats*
¼	cup ground flaxseed meal
¼	cup shredded unsweetened coconut
1	teaspoon ground cinnamon
¼	teaspoon ground ginger
¼	teaspoon ground nutmeg
¼	teaspoon sea salt
¼	cup honey
½	cup cashew or almond butter
½	cup finely chopped dried apricots
¼	cup unsweetened dried cranberries or goji berries

1. Preheat the oven to 350°F. Coat an 8" x 8" square baking pan with canola oil cooking spray.

2. Combine the oats, flaxseed, coconut, cinnamon, ginger, nutmeg, and salt in a large bowl.

3. Combine the honey and cashew butter in a small bowl. Pour into the dry ingredients and stir to combine. Stir in the apricots and cranberries until well combined.

4. Press the mixture firmly into the pan. Bake for 25 minutes, or until the edges are browned.

5. Let cool completely before cutting into 8 bars. Serve with 1 cup of fat-free milk. Store in an airtight container up to 1 week.

Makes 8 servings

* Use oats labeled gluten-free.

Lunch

Quick Quesadilla & Guac with Black Bean Salad

`GF`

Black Bean Salad

- ½ cup canned black beans, rinsed and drained
- ¼ cup chopped grape tomatoes
- 1 tablespoon chunky salsa
- 1 tablespoon finely chopped shallot or red onion
- 1 tablespoon finely chopped cilantro
- 1 teaspoon lime juice

Quesadilla and Guacamole

- 2 6″ corn tortillas
- 2 tablespoons shredded Monterey Jack or Cheddar cheese
- 2 slices (2 ounces) roasted turkey breast (such as Applegate Naturals)
- ¼ Hass avocado
- 2 teaspoons finely chopped shallot
- 1 teaspoon lime juice
- 1 tablespoon fat-free plain Greek yogurt

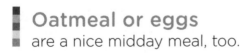

Oatmeal or eggs
are a nice midday meal, too.

1. To make the salad: Combine the beans, tomatoes, salsa, shallot, cilantro, and lime juice in small bowl. Season with salt and freshly ground black pepper to taste. Set aside.

2. To make the quesadilla: Coat a small nonstick skillet with canola oil cooking spray and place over medium heat.

3. Place one tortilla in the skillet and sprinkle it with 1 tablespoon of cheese. Lay the turkey flat on top of the cheese and sprinkle the remaining 1 tablespoon of cheese on top. Place the other tortilla on top. Cook the quesadilla for 2 minutes per side, or until the tortillas are slightly browned and the cheese is melted. Flip gently, keeping the tortillas in place.

4. To make the guacamole: Mash the avocado in a small bowl with a fork and stir in the shallot and lime juice.

5. Cut the quesadilla into quarters and top it with the yogurt and the guacamole. Serve it with the black bean salad.

Redefine your idea
of "setback" or "failure."
Remember: Every meal is Monday morning!

Quinoa Pasta Primavera

`GF` `VEG`

- 2 teaspoons extra-virgin olive oil
- 1 zucchini, cut into ⅛"-thick rounds and halved
- ⅓ cup chopped red bell pepper, cut into 1" pieces
- ¼ cup frozen corn or sweet peas, thawed
- ½ teaspoon minced garlic
- ½ cup hot cooked quinoa-blend pasta (such as Ancient Harvest)
- 3 tablespoons freshly grated Parmesan cheese
- 1 tablespoon finely chopped fresh basil

1. Heat 1 teaspoon of the oil in a large nonstick skillet over medium heat.

2. Add the zucchini and pepper and season with salt and freshly ground black pepper to taste. Cook for 7 minutes, stirring occasionally, or until the vegetables are softened and the zucchini is slightly golden.

3. Reduce the heat to medium-low. Stir in the corn and garlic and cook for 2 more minutes.

4. Transfer the vegetable mixture to a bowl, add the pasta, and toss with the cheese, basil, and the remaining 1 teaspoon of oil.

Go meatless

Pick a day this week to skip meat in your meals and see how you feel. Vegetarians tend to eat 200 fewer calories per day.

Waldorf-Style Chicken Salad with Balsamic Dressing

`GF` `NC`

4	(2 ounces) precooked frozen grilled chicken strips (such as FreeBird)
2	cups baby spinach
2	tablespoons (1 ounce) soft goat cheese, crumbled
2	teaspoons dried cranberries
1	tablespoon chopped walnuts
½	cup chopped Granny Smith apple
2	teaspoons balsamic vinegar
1	teaspoon grapeseed oil

1. Microwave the chicken according to package directions and cut into a ½" dice.

2. Combine the chicken, spinach, goat cheese, cranberries, walnuts, and apple in a bowl and toss with the vinegar and oil.

Protein power
Vow to eat a different protein today than your usual, to avoid a plan rut.

Tuna Tabbouleh

`GF` `VEG` `NC`

2   teaspoons lemon juice
2   teaspoons cold-pressed olive oil
1   teaspoon red wine vinegar
1   can (5 ounces) chunk light tuna packed in water, drained
⅓   cup cooked quinoa, cooled to room temperature
¼   cup grape tomatoes, cut into quarters
¼   cup peeled and chopped cucumber
1   tablespoon finely chopped fresh parsley
½   cup sliced cucumber
2   tablespoons hummus

1. Stir the lemon juice, olive oil, and red wine vinegar in a small bowl and set aside.

2. Break the tuna into chunks using a fork and combine with the quinoa, tomatoes, chopped cucumber, and parsley in another bowl.

3. Add the reserved dressing to the quinoa mixture and toss to combine. Season with salt and freshly ground black pepper to taste.

4. Serve with the sliced cucumber and hummus on the side.

Find yourself a farmer
Go to localharvest.org and enter your ZIP code to find your nearest community-supported agriculture (CSA) options.

Baby Spinach & Artichoke Salad

`GF` `VEG` `NC`

2	teaspoons lemon juice
2	teaspoons red wine vinegar
1	teaspoon cold-pressed olive oil
¼	teaspoon minced garlic
¼	teaspoon dried oregano
2	cups baby spinach
½	cup canned quartered artichoke hearts, drained
½	cup canned white beans, rinsed and drained
⅓	cup grape tomatoes, cut into quarters
2	tablespoons freshly grated Parmesan cheese

1. Combine the lemon juice, vinegar, oil, garlic, and oregano in a small bowl. Set aside.

2. Toss the spinach, artichoke hearts, beans, tomatoes, and cheese in another bowl.

3. Add the reserved dressing to the spinach mixture and stir to combine.

Boil a few eggs
and keep them in your fridge for easy snacking. (But toss them after 1 week—boiled eggs are more vulnerable to bacteria than fresh ones.)

Peanut-Tofu Lettuce Cups

4	leaves Boston or Bibb lettuce
1	teaspoon natural crunchy peanut butter
2	teaspoons honey
1	teaspoon sesame oil
¼	teaspoon grated ginger
4	ounces firm tofu, cut into ½" dice
½	cup chopped cucumber
½	cup grated carrot
2	tablespoons thinly sliced scallion

1. Place the lettuce leaves in a single layer on a serving plate.

2. Combine the peanut butter, honey, oil, and ginger in a small bowl. Set aside.

3. Toss the tofu, cucumber, carrot, and scallion in another bowl. Season with salt and freshly ground black pepper to taste.

4. Divide the tofu mixture among the lettuce leaves. Drizzle the reserved peanut-ginger sauce on top.

Chopathon

Spend 20 minutes in the kitchen prechopping vegetables, including carrots, celery, peppers, and onions, to make cooking and snacking easier throughout the week.

Sweet & Salty Beet Salad

`GF` `VEG` `NC`

- 1   tablespoon plus 2 teaspoons fig or balsamic vinegar
- 1   tablespoon finely chopped shallot
- 1   teaspoon finely chopped fresh thyme or $\frac{1}{2}$ teaspoon dried
- 2   cups baby arugula
- $\frac{1}{3}$ cup canned, prepackaged, or fresh beets, peeled and thinly sliced into half-moons
- 1   small plum, thinly sliced into half-moons
- 1   tablespoon chopped pistachios
- $\frac{1}{2}$ ounce crumbled goat cheese

1. Combine the vinegar, shallot, and thyme in a small bowl. Season with salt and freshly ground black pepper to taste. Set aside.

2. Place the arugula, beets, plum, pistachios, and goat cheese in another bowl. Add the reserved dressing and toss to combine. Serve with 4 multigrain crackers.

Drink a liquid lunch
Even if you're not usually a smoothie fan, try one, just to see how it strikes you. Most people say smoothies satisfy them for hours.

Plum-Dandy Sandwich

GF* VEG NC

    1 medium plum
  ³⁄₄ cup (6 ounces) plain nonfat yogurt
    1 teaspoon honey
  ¹⁄₄ teaspoon ground cinnamon
    2 teaspoons smooth or chunky nut butter
    1 slice multigrain bread, toasted*

1. Cut two ¹⁄₈"-thick rounds off one side of the plum. Set aside. Chop the remaining plum into small pieces and place them in a small bowl.

2. Add the yogurt to the bowl and stir in ¹⁄₂ teaspoon of the honey and ¹⁄₈ teaspoon of the cinnamon until combined.

3. Spread the nut butter on the toast and sprinkle it with the remaining ¹⁄₈ teaspoon cinnamon. Place the reserved plum slices flat on top of the bread and drizzle with the remaining ¹⁄₂ teaspoon honey. Serve with the yogurt mixture on the side.

* Use gluten-free whole-grain bread.

Write down a list
of produce you want to eat this week. People who commit to a concrete plan to eat more fruits and vegetables are twice as likely to stick with that plan.

Salmon, Lentil & Cucumber Salad

GF VEG NC

2	teaspoons balsamic vinegar
½	teaspoon cold-pressed olive oil
½	teaspoon minced garlic
¼	teaspoon dried oregano
½	cup canned lentils, rinsed and drained, or precooked lentils
¼	cup finely chopped cucumber
¼	cup finely chopped or shredded carrot
¼	cup chopped red bell pepper
2	tablespoons minced scallions
1	can (3.75 ounces) salmon, drained, or leftover cooked salmon, chunked

1. Combine the vinegar, oil, garlic, and oregano in a small bowl. Set aside.

2. Combine the lentils, cucumber, carrot, pepper, and scallions in another bowl. Toss with the reserved dressing.

3. Add the salmon and gently toss to combine. Season with salt and freshly ground black pepper to taste.

Dinner

Veggie Burger with Purple Potato Salad

`VEG` `NC`

- ½ cup baby purple creamer potatoes (3 to 4 potatoes)
- ½ cup frozen broccoli florets
- 1 tablespoon finely chopped fresh basil
- 1 tablespoon finely chopped fresh parsley
- 1 tablespoon lemon juice
- 1 teaspoon cold-pressed olive oil
- ½ teaspoon minced garlic
- 1½ teaspoons Dijon mustard
- 1 frozen veggie burger (such as Amy's California Veggie Burger)
- ½ cup baby arugula
- 1 tablespoon plain hummus (such as Tribe)

Chew more!

People who chew each bite 40 times eat 12 percent less than those who chew 15 times or fewer.

1. Pierce the potatoes on all sides with a fork. Microwave for 3 to 5 minutes, or until softened. Let stand to cool to room temperature.

2. Microwave the broccoli according to package directions and let stand to cool to room temperature.

3. Combine the basil, parsley, lemon juice, oil, garlic, and $\frac{1}{2}$ teaspoon of the mustard in a small bowl. Season with salt and freshly ground black pepper to taste. Set aside.

4. Microwave the veggie burger according to package directions. Cut the potatoes into quarters when cool and toss with the broccoli and 2 teaspoons of the reserved dressing.

5. Toss the arugula with the remaining dressing and transfer to a serving dish. Place the veggie burger on top.

6. Combine the hummus with the remaining 1 teaspoon mustard in a small bowl and serve on top of the veggie burger with potato salad on the side.

Ask around at work

for a new weight loss buddy. You don't need someone to do the plan with you (although that's a great idea!). But finding someone you can brag to a little about your successes—or confess to when you've had a setback—will provide solid support.

Roasted Portobello Stack with Chili-Spiced Sweet Potato Wedges

1   small sweet potato, cut into $\frac{1}{2}$"-thick wedges
2   teaspoons grapeseed oil
$\frac{1}{4}$ teaspoon ground cumin plus a dash
$\frac{1}{4}$ teaspoon chili powder or ground paprika plus a dash
1   tablespoon lemon juice
$1\frac{1}{2}$ teaspoons Dijon mustard
1   teaspoon minced garlic
1   portobello mushroom cap
$\frac{1}{2}$ cup sliced sweet onion, cut in $\frac{1}{4}$"-thick slices
1   slice (1 ounce) Cheddar cheese
2   tablespoons fat-free plain yogurt

1. Preheat the oven to 425°F. Coat a baking sheet with canola oil cooking spray.

2. Toss the sweet potato with 1 teaspoon of the oil, $\frac{1}{4}$ teaspoon cumin, and $\frac{1}{4}$ teaspoon paprika to coat in a large bowl. Season with salt and freshly ground black pepper. Place on the

▌Brush your teeth
▪ right after dinner, to curb evening eating.

baking sheet in a single layer and bake for 25 minutes, flipping halfway through.

3. Make the marinade by mixing $\frac{1}{2}$ teaspoon of the remaining oil, a dash of cumin, 2 teaspoons of the lemon juice, $\frac{1}{2}$ teaspoon of the mustard, and $\frac{1}{2}$ teaspoon of the garlic in a small bowl. Place the mushroom in a resealable plastic bag and pour the marinade on top. Seal and toss to coat.

4. Heat the remaining $\frac{1}{2}$ teaspoon oil in a small nonstick skillet over low heat. Add the onions and cover. Cook for 6 to 8 minutes, stirring once, until the onion is translucent. Increase the heat to medium and cook for another 10 to 12 minutes, uncovered, until the onion is well browned.

5. After the sweet potatoes have cooked for 25 minutes, flip them and move them to one side of the baking sheet. Discard the excess marinade from the mushroom, place it on the opposite side of the baking sheet, and season it with salt and freshly ground black pepper. Bake for 10 minutes, or until the mushroom is tender and the potato wedges are browned.

6. Place the cheese on top of the mushroom and bake for 1 to 2 more minutes, or until the cheese is melted.

7. Combine the yogurt with the remaining 1 teaspoon mustard, the remaining $\frac{1}{2}$ teaspoon garlic, the remaining lemon juice, and a dash of paprika.

8. Top the mushroom with the onion slices, and serve with the sweet potato wedges and the yogurt dipping sauce on the side.

Roasting rocks
Resolve to try one roasted vegetable this week.
You'll thank me forever.

Parmesan-Coated Halibut & Spicy Sprouts

GF VEG

1 cup brussels sprouts, trimmed and halved
1 teaspoon cold-pressed olive oil
1 (4 ounce) skinless wild halibut filet, about ½" thick
2 tablespoons grated Parmesan cheese
¼ teaspoon dried oregano
1 lemon wedge
¼ teaspoon chili pepper flakes

1. Preheat the oven to 400°F. Lightly mist a baking dish with canola oil cooking spray and set aside.

2. Toss the brussels sprouts in a small bowl with the oil. Season with salt and freshly ground black pepper. Place in a single layer in the baking dish and bake for 20 minutes.

3. Combine cheese and oregano in a shallow dish. Lightly mist fish on both sides with canola oil spray and dredge each side in cheese mixture. Season with salt and freshly ground black pepper. Refrigerate until ready for use.

4. Reduce the oven temperature to 375°F. Flip the sprouts and move them to one side of the baking dish. Add the fish on the opposite side of the dish and bake for 10 minutes, or until the fish is opaque throughout.

5. Combine the remaining 1 tablespoon of cheese and the oregano in a shallow dish and sprinkle it over the fish. Squeeze the lemon wedge over the sprouts and toss with chili pepper flakes before serving.

Creamy Thai
Sweet Potato Bisque

`GF` `VEG`

1	teaspoon grapeseed or cold-pressed olive oil
¼	cup chopped sweet or yellow onion
1	cup almond or rice milk
1	medium sweet potato, peeled and cut into 1″ chunks
2	sprigs cilantro plus 1 tablespoon chopped
1	teaspoon smooth peanut butter
¼	teaspoon minced ginger
¼	teaspoon ground curry powder
2	teaspoons unsweetened shredded coconut

1. Heat the oil over medium heat in a small saucepan. Cook the onion over medium-high heat for 3 minutes, or until softened. Transfer to a blender or food processor fitted with a metal blade.

2. Lightly coat the same pan with canola oil cooking spray and place over medium-low heat.

3. Add the milk, sweet potato, and cilantro springs to the pan. Cover and simmer 15 minutes, or until the potatoes are tender, stirring halfway through.

4. Remove the pan from the heat and let cool for 10 minutes. Discard the cilantro sprigs. Transfer the potato and milk to the blender with the onion and puree until smooth.

5. Return the potato mixture to the pan. Stir in the peanut butter, ginger, curry powder, and chopped cilantro. Season with salt and freshly ground black pepper to taste. Cook over low heat for 1 to 2 minutes until heated through. Serve garnished with the coconut.

Arugula, Prosciutto & Parmesan Salad

`GF` `NC`

2 teaspoons fig vinegar
1 teaspoon cold-pressed olive or grapeseed oil
2 thin slices prosciutto
1½ cups baby arugula
3 tablespoons shaved Parmigiano-Reggiano or Parmesan cheese
8 hazelnuts, halved
1 Black Mission fig, cut into quarters

1. Combine the vinegar and oil in a small bowl. Set aside.

2. Arrange the prosciutto flat on a serving plate.

3. Place the arugula, cheese, and hazelnuts in another bowl and toss to combine. Season with salt and freshly ground black pepper to taste.

4. Spoon the arugula mixture on top of the prosciutto and drizzle with the reserved syrup mixture. Serve garnished with the fig.

Twice the spice

Next time you're shopping, grab a spice you've never tried and find a recipe to test-drive it.

Jambalaya-Style Stir-Fry

`GF` `VEG`

  1 teaspoon cold-pressed olive oil
 ½ cup thinly sliced celery (about 2 stalks)
 ⅓ cup finely chopped onion
 ¼ cup chopped green bell pepper
 ½ cup chopped tomato
  1 teaspoon minced garlic
  1 tablespoon chopped fresh parsley
Dash of ground cloves
Dash of dried oregano
Dash of ground red pepper (optional)
  8 (3 ounces) wild rock or small shrimp, shelled and deveined
 ⅓ cup hot cooked black or brown rice

1. Place the oil in a large nonstick skillet over medium heat. Add the celery, onion, and pepper and season with salt and freshly ground black pepper. Cook for 5 to 7 minutes, or until vegetables are slightly softened.

2. Stir in the tomato, garlic, parsley, cloves, oregano, and ground red pepper (if using). Reduce the heat to medium low and cook for 2 minutes.

3. Add the shrimp to the pan and cook for 5 more minutes, or until the shrimp is opaque throughout. Serve immediately over the rice.

Bored?
Try "brinner," a nickname for "breakfast for dinner."

Crunchy Caesar Salad with Grilled Chicken

`GF` `NC`

- ⅓ cup fat-free plain yogurt
- 1 teaspoon minced garlic
- 1 teaspoon Dijon mustard
- 2 teaspoons lemon juice
- ¾ teaspoon Worcestershire sauce
- 4 to 5 ounces boneless, skinless chicken breast (about ¾" thick)
- 1 teaspoon pine nuts
- 2 cups chopped romaine lettuce hearts
- 2 tablespoons freshly grated Parmesan cheese

1. Combine the yogurt, garlic, mustard, lemon juice, and Worcestershire sauce in a small bowl. Season with salt and freshly ground black pepper. Reserve and refrigerate 2 tablespoons of the yogurt mixture.

Go on a color quest at the farmers' market
Try to score at least seven fruits and vegetables of different colors.

2. Place the chicken in a bowl with the remaining yogurt mixture, tossing to coat. Cover and marinate the chicken for at least 15 minutes, or up to 2 hours.

3. Place a small nonstick skillet over medium heat. Add the pine nuts and toast, stirring frequently, for 3 minutes, or until lightly browned and fragrant. Set aside.

4. When you're ready to cook the chicken, coat the skillet with canola oil cooking spray and return to medium heat. Using a fork, remove the chicken from the bowl and shake off and discard the excess marinade. Season with salt and freshly ground black pepper. Place the chicken in the skillet and cook for 6 minutes per side, or until cooked through, turning to ensure doneness on all sides. Let the chicken stand for 5 minutes before cutting into 1" pieces.

5. Combine the lettuce, cheese, and the reserved pine nuts in a bowl. Add the reserved yogurt mixture and the chicken, tossing to coat. Serve immediately.

Romance your raspberries

Pick one food you'll eat today, and promise yourself you'll eat this one food slowly, joyfully, and mindfully. Mindful eating has been shown to help people consume 300 fewer calories per day.

Greek Pita Pizza & Two-Step Spinach Sauté

VEG

2   slices tomato, ⅛" thick
2   mini whole-wheat pitas
2   tablespoons (1 ounce) crumbled feta cheese
6   black olives, cut into quarters
1   tablespoon minced shallot or red onion
2   teaspoons cold-pressed olive oil
¼   teaspoon dried oregano
3   cups baby spinach
½   teaspoon minced garlic

1. Preheat the oven to 400°F. Line a baking sheet with parchment paper.

2. Place 1 tomato slice flat on top of each pita. Divide the cheese, olives, and shallot on top of the tomatoes and drizzle pitas with 1 teaspoon of the oil. Sprinkle with the oregano and season with freshly ground black pepper to taste.

3. Place the pitas on the baking sheet and bake 12 to 15 minutes, or until the edges are slightly browned.

4. Place the remaining 1 teaspoon oil in a small nonstick skillet over medium heat. Add the spinach and garlic and season with salt and freshly ground black pepper. Cook, stirring occasionally, for about 3 minutes, or until the spinach is just wilted. Serve the spinach on the side of the pita pizza.

Tuna-Stuffed Tomato

1   large beefsteak or heirloom tomato
½   cup canned cannellini beans, rinsed and drained
½   cup canned quartered artichoke hearts, drained,
    or frozen and thawed, chopped
¼   cup finely chopped shallot or red onion
2   tablespoons chopped fresh basil
2   teaspoons cold-pressed olive oil
1½ teaspoons red wine vinegar
3   ounces chunk light tuna packed in water, drained

1. Cut the top off the tomato and set the top aside.
Gently hollow out the tomato, leaving ¼" on the bottom and
side. Set the tomato shell aside. Discard the juice and seeds
from the interior flesh and chop the flesh into small pieces.

2. Place the chopped flesh in a bowl. Add the beans, ¼ cup
of the artichokes, 2 tablespoons of the shallot, 1 tablespoon of
the basil, 1 teaspoon of the oil, and ½ teaspoon of the vinegar.
Toss to combine. Season with salt and freshly ground black
pepper to taste.

3. Place the tuna in a separate small bowl. Add the remaining
¼ cup artichokes, 2 tablespoons shallot, 1 tablespoon basil,
1 teaspoon oil, and 1 teaspoon vinegar and toss to combine.
Season with salt and freshly ground black pepper to taste.

4. Spoon the tuna mixture into the reserved tomato shell and
cover with the reserved top. Serve with the bean salad on
the side.

The New You and Improved Meal Plan

Ready to get started? Here are a few quick tips.

Every day, drink at least 2 cups of green tea. The antioxidants are great for your health and also speed weight loss. Also, drink at least 8 glasses of water.

Every night with dinner, have a salad of at least 1 cup of greens—spinach, kale, and mesclun are all great—in addition to the veggie you're having. If you have prepared your evening meal with an oil, eat your salad greens with vinegar, herbs, spices, or lemon juice. For example, on your Burger to Bite night, you won't need to add a fat. But if you skip the cheese, go ahead and get your fat serving either by having a tablespoon of oil-based dressing, a portion of nuts, or 2 teaspoons of oil.

Add as many herbs and spices as you like. I didn't want to intimidate you by using so many different ingredients in each meal, but these really ratchet up the flavor and nutrition level of everything you eat. Cinnamon, nutmeg, cloves, oregano, thyme, rosemary, basil, and parsley are always on my countertop. Experiment with parsley on your cucumber salad and nutmeg in your cottage cheese. Aim to add some to every meal and snack!

New You and Improved Cooking Tips

BAKING In general, whole cuts of meat such as beef and pork should be cooked until a food thermometer inserted in the thickest part of the meat reaches an internal temperature of at least 145°F, or 160°F for ground meat. All poultry items should reach 165°F. All meat should rest for 3 minutes after cooking to ensure doneness. Fish should be baked until it is opaque throughout, reaches 145°F, and flakes easily with a fork. Whole potatoes should be pierced with a fork and baked at 400°F for 45 minutes or until tender, depending on size.

BOILING Generally, grains can be simmered covered, until water is absorbed and grains are softened, using a 1:2 grains to water ratio and a dash of salt. Turn off the heat and let rest for a few minutes before stirring.

GRILLING Coat a nonstick pan with canola oil spray and place over medium-high heat. Season meat and seafood with sea salt and pepper before grilling.

ROASTING For no-fuss roasting, mist veggies with 3 sprays canola oil spray, toss and spread in a single layer on a baking sheet. Roast at 400°F for 15 minutes, turning once. For "burnt" veggies, place in a roasting pan, drizzle with olive oil, season with kosher salt and pepper, and bake at 375°F for 40 minutes or until edges look black. For chicken and most meats, coat on all sides with 1 tsp olive oil, and season with sea salt and pepper. Place in baking pan and roast at 400°F for 20 minutes or until cooked through (see temperatures above for baking).

SAUTEING AND STIR-FRYING Coat a nonstick skillet with canola oil spray and cook meat first, then remove from skillet. Coat the pan once more with spray and add veggies. Cook veggies until fork-tender, then add meat and mix with a dash of soy sauce or seasoning as indicated. (Remember to peel and devein shrimp!)

WEEK 1: **Eat More, Not Less**

	Monday	Tuesday	Wednesday
Breakfast	**Simple Scrambled Eggs** 1 whole egg plus 2 egg whites (scrambled) ½ tsp dried oregano	**Simple Scrambled Eggs** 1 whole egg plus 2 egg whites (scrambled) ½ tsp dried oregano	**Simple Scrambled Eggs** 1 whole egg plus 2 egg whites (scrambled) ½ tsp dried oregano
Snack 1	1 medium Granny Smith apple ½ tsp ground cinnamon	1 medium Granny Smith apple ½ tsp ground cinnamon	1 medium Granny Smith apple ½ tsp ground cinnamon
Lunch	**Lentil Spinach Salad** Spinach ½ cup cooked lentils 1 hard-boiled egg 2 tsp olive oil	**Lentil Spinach Salad** Spinach ½ cup cooked lentils 1 hard-boiled egg 2 tsp olive oil	**Lentil Spinach Salad** Spinach ½ cup cooked lentils 1 hard-boiled egg 2 tsp olive oil
Snack 2	½ cup artichoke hearts *or* 1 small steamed artichoke with a squeeze of lemon	½ cup artichoke hearts *or* 1 small steamed artichoke with a squeeze of lemon	½ cup artichoke hearts *or* 1 small steamed artichoke with a squeeze of lemon
Dinner	**Salmon Spinach Salad** Spinach 4 oz salmon (grilled/broiled) ¼ avocado	**Salmon Spinach Salad** Spinach 4 oz salmon (grilled/broiled) ¼ avocado	**Salmon Spinach Salad** Spinach 4 oz salmon (grilled/broiled) ¼ avocado

Thursday	Friday	Saturday	Sunday
Simple Scrambled Eggs 1 whole egg plus 2 egg whites (scrambled) ½ tsp dried oregano	**Going Grainy** ⅓ cup cooked quinoa or oatmeal 1 hard-boiled egg Black pepper (to taste)	**Going Grainy** ⅓ cup cooked quinoa or oatmeal 1 hard-boiled egg Black pepper (to taste)	**Going Grainy** ⅓ cup cooked quinoa or oatmeal 1 hard-boiled egg Black pepper (to taste)
1 medium Granny Smith apple ½ tsp ground cinnamon	1 medium Granny Smith apple 2 tsp peanut butter ½ tsp ground cinnamon	1 medium Granny Smith apple 2 tsp peanut butter ½ tsp ground cinnamon	1 medium Granny Smith apple 2 tsp peanut butter ½ tsp ground cinnamon
Lentil Spinach Salad Spinach ½ cup cooked lentils 1 hard-boiled egg 2 tsp olive oil	**Chicken Spinach Salad** Spinach 4 oz chicken (grilled/broiled) ¼ avocado	**Shrimp Spinach Salad** Spinach 4 oz shrimp (grilled/broiled) ¼ avocado	**Turkey Spinach Salad** Spinach 4 oz sliced deli turkey ¼ avocado
½ cup artichoke hearts or 1 small steamed artichoke with a squeeze of lemon	½ cup artichoke hearts or 1 small steamed artichoke with a squeeze of lemon or 6 oz fat-free plain Greek yogurt	½ cup artichoke hearts or 1 small steamed artichoke with a squeeze of lemon or 6 oz fat-free plain Greek yogurt	½ cup artichoke hearts or 1 small steamed artichoke with a squeeze of lemon or 6 oz fat-free plain Greek yogurt
Salmon Spinach Salad 4 oz salmon (grilled/broiled) Spinach ¼ avocado	**Cod Cleanse** 4 oz cod (broiled) Broccoli (steamed) 2 tsp olive oil	**Chicken Spinach Salad** 4 oz chicken Spinach ¼ avocado	**Pork Tenderloin & Bok Choy** 4 oz pork tenderloin (grilled) Bok choy (steamed) 2 tsp olive oil

WEEK 1: **Eat More, Not Less**

Got a craving but not sure you're hungry? Set your smartphone timer for 10 minutes and distract yourself. If you're still hungry when it goes off, fix yourself an appealing snack.

VISUALIZE YOUR SUCCESS BY PUTTING A PICTURE OF SOMETHING YOU WANT—A PRETTY NEW DRESS IN A SMALLER SIZE, FOR EXAMPLE—ON YOUR FRIDGE.

You're just starting the plan. What do you miss? Baked goods? A martini? If you're not craving anything, great. But if you are, make a plan to have a conscious indulgence next week. Just wait; you probably won't even want it.

Double-check your food journal. While keeping a food journal has been proven to help people almost double their weight loss, it's easy to get sloppy as the weeks go by. Solidify good habits now.

Facing a big meal out? Whether it's a holiday at a relative's or a supertempting restaurant, researchers say downing two glasses of water before sitting down to eat means you'll consume between 75 and 90 fewer calories at the meal.

Snack stronger: Controlled snacks will reduce your chancesof overeating later in the day. Be prepared!

TAKE IT UP A NOTCH AND BE EXTRA VIGILANT ON WEEKENDS, SINCE PEOPLE TEND TO OVEREAT ON THESE DAYS—ABOUT 115 CALORIES PER DAY MORE, ON AVERAGE— THAN ON WEEKDAYS.

WEEK 2: **Breathe Your Way Thin**

	Monday	Tuesday	Wednesday
Breakfast	**Savory Oatmeal** ⅓ cup cooked oatmeal 2 oz part-skim ricotta cheese 3 Tbsp grated Parmesan cheese Black pepper (to taste)	**Simple Scrambled Eggs** 1 whole egg plus 2 egg whites (scrambled) ½ tsp dried oregano	**Quinoa Crunch** ⅓ cup cooked quinoa 6 oz fat-free plain Greek yogurt 1 Tbsp chia seeds
Snack 1	8 cashews Celery sticks	8 cashews Celery sticks	8 cashews Celery sticks
Lunch	**Crrrrunch Salad** 2 cups baby spinach 1 cup sliced cucumber 10 strips yellow bell pepper ½ cup chickpeas 18 pistachios 4 crumbled fiber crackers	**Salmon Spinach Salad** Spinach 4 oz salmon (grilled/broiled) ¼ avocado	**Lentil Salad** 2 cups arugula ½ cup cherry tomatoes ¼ cup diced red onion ½ cup cooked lentils 2 tsp olive oil
Snack 2	6 oz fat-free plain Greek yogurt 2 Tbsp flaxseed	**Green Tea Latte** 1 cup green tea plus 1 cup steamed soy or almond milk	6 oz fat-free plain Greek yogurt 2 Tbsp flaxseed
Dinner	**Shrimp Marinara** 4 oz shrimp (steamed) ½ cup marinara sauce Burnt veggies (see page 197) 1 tsp capers 2 tsp olive oil	**Cod Cleanse** 4 oz cod (broiled) Broccoli (steamed) 2 tsp olive oil	**Burger to Bite** 4 oz 85% lean organic ground beef burger Mashed cauliflower 1 oz Cheddar

Thursday	Friday	Saturday	Sunday
Going Grainy ⅓ cup cooked quinoa or oatmeal 1 hard-boiled egg Black pepper (to taste)	**Caprese Breakfast** 1 slice Ezekiel bread (toasted) 1 slice tomato 1 oz low-fat mozzarella cheese 2 tsp olive oil	**Simple Scrambled Eggs** 1 whole egg plus 2 egg whites (scrambled) ½ tsp dried oregano	**Keri's Favorite Smoothie** 1 small banana 1 cup almond milk 1 tsp almond butter ⅛ avocado 1 cup ice
8 cashews Celery sticks	8 cashews Carrot sticks	8 cashews Carrot sticks	8 cashews Carrot sticks
Chicken Spinach Salad Spinach 4 oz chicken (grilled/broiled) ¼ avocado	**Mini Roasted Veggie Wraps** 10 strips red bell pepper ¼ cup grilled zucchini ¼ cup grilled eggplant 3 oz low-fat feta cheese 2 tsp olive oil 2 small corn tortillas	**Salmon Spinach Salad** Spinach 4 oz salmon (grilled/broiled) ¼ avocado	**Antipasto Platter** 2 Tbsp roasted red bell peppers 4 Tbsp hummus 1 oz low-fat feta cheese or 12 large olives 4 fiber crackers
Green Tea Latte 1 cup green tea plus 1 cup steamed soy or almond milk	6 oz fat-free plain Greek yogurt 2 Tbsp flaxseed	**Green Tea Latte** 1 cup green tea plus 1 cup steamed soy or almond milk	6 oz fat-free plain Greek yogurt 2 Tbsp flaxseed
Parmesan-Coated Halibut & Spicy Sprouts See page 188.	**Chicken Spinach Salad** Spinach 4 oz chicken (grilled/broiled) ¼ avocado	**Pork Tenderloin & Bok Choy** 4 oz pork tenderloin (grilled) Bok choy (steamed) 2 tsp olive oil	**Steak & Sautéed Spinach** 4 oz steak (grilled) 2 cups spinach (sautéed) 2 tsp olive oil

WEEK 2: **Breathe Your Way Thin**

Add mellow music to your iPod, and listen to something more soothing—classical, jazz, or whatever—than your usual choices for at least 5 minutes.

Commuting is typically one of the most stressful parts of the day. Do something radical to shake yours up: Download an audiobook, leave a half hour earlier, drive a new route.

TRY DOING A GUIDED MEDITATION THAT YOU'VE DOWNLOADED, TO SEE HOW IT FEELS. SITES LIKE BELIEFNET.ORG CAN GET YOU STARTED; UCLA (MARC. UCLA.EDU/BODY.CFM?ID=22) ALSO OFFERS SOME EXCELLENT FREE DOWNLOADS.

Use waiting—at the bank, in the dentist's office, as your computer boots up—to practice a few moments of conscious breathing.

Load a "happy place" picture onto your desktop, such as a photo of a favorite place or a loved one, or even a serene spot you like to imagine yourself in.

Sniff out serenity: Keep a bottle of an essential oil on your desk and take a whiff now and again. (I like lavender.)

We're assaulted by sound, but we can control some of the noise. Whether it's a ring tone or your morning alarm, switch it to something more soothing, like chimes or raindrops.

IRON: SERIOUSLY, RHYTHMIC HOUSEWORK, WHICH ALSO INCLUDES CHOPPING VEGETABLES AND MOPPING, CAN BECOME MEDITATIVE IF YOU GO SLOW AND BREATHE DEEPLY.

Give yourself time to stress. Instead of telling yourself to "stop worrying already" (like that ever works!), set aside a certain amount of time to sit down and stew about your problem—let's say you decide on 10 minutes after dinner. If you catch yourself worrying before or after, remind yourself you *can* worry about it, just not right now.

Be present in the moment: If you catch yourself multitasking, strip the activities down until you are focused on just one thing, and do it mindfully. While some new research indicates that multitasking may not be as brain-circuit jamming as we once thought and may actually help us concentrate, it's still a good mindfulness practice to occasionally zero in on a single task.

WEEK 3: Sip Your Way Slim

	Monday	Tuesday	Wednesday
Breakfast	**Monday Morning Detox** See page 163.	**Simple Scrambled Eggs** 1 whole egg plus 2 egg whites (scrambled) ½ tsp dried oregano	**Quinoa Crunch** ⅓ cup cooked quinoa 6 oz fat-free plain Greek yogurt 1 Tbsp chia seeds
Snack 1	**Greens Juice** Kale, celery, romaine, cucumber lemon, ginger, with ¼ avocado *or* 10 almonds	Celery sticks 1 oz low-fat goat cheese	**Greens Juice** Kale, celery, romaine, cucumber, lemon, ginger, with ¼ avocado *or* 10 almonds
Lunch	**Turkey Salad** 2 cups chopped endive ½ cup cherry tomatoes 4 oz sliced deli turkey 2 tsp olive oil Balsamic vinegar (to taste)	**Salmon Spinach Salad** Spinach 4 oz salmon (grilled/broiled) ¼ avocado	**Crrrrunch Salad** 2 cups baby spinach 1 cup sliced cucumber 10 strips yellow bell pepper ½ cup chickpeas 18 pistachios 4 crumbled fiber crackers
Snack 2	**Raspberry Smoothie** 1 cup almond milk 1 cup raspberries 2 tsp almond butter	6 oz fat-free plain Greek yogurt 1 Tbsp pumpkin seeds	**Raspberry Smoothie** 1 cup almond milk 1 cup raspberries 2 tsp almond butter
Dinner	**Lentil Spinach Salad & Chicken** 4 oz chicken (grilled/broiled) Spinach ½ cup cooked lentils 2 tsp olive oil	**Pork Tenderloin & Bok Choy** 4 oz pork tenderloin (grilled) Bok choy (steamed) 2 tsp olive oil	**Tofu Kebabs & Spinach** 4 oz firm tofu, cubed and alternated on skewer with red and yellow peppers, red onions, mushrooms 1 cup spinach (steamed) 2 tsp toasted sesame oil

Thursday	Friday	Saturday	Sunday
Keri's Favorite Smoothie 1 small banana 1 cup almond milk 1 tsp almond butter ⅛ avocado 1 cup ice	**Going Grainy** ⅓ cup cooked quinoa or oatmeal 1 hard-boiled egg ½ tsp black pepper	**Simple Scrambled Eggs** 1 whole egg plus 2 egg whites (scrambled) ½ tsp dried oregano	**Awesome Avocado** 1 slice Ezekiel bread (toasted) ½ cup fat-free cottage cheese ¼ avocado
Celery sticks 1 oz low-fat goat cheese	**Greens Juice** Kale, celery, romaine, cucumber, lemon, ginger, with ¼ avocado *or* 10 almonds	Celery sticks 1 oz low-fat goat cheese	**Greens Juice** Kale, celery, romaine, cucumber, lemon, ginger, with ¼ avocado *or* 10 almonds
Slim Slaw with Shrimp ½ cup sliced red cabbage ½ cup sliced green cabbage 4 oz grilled shrimp 10 sliced almonds 1 Tbsp rice vinegar 1 tsp Dijon mustard	**Shrimp Spinach Salad** Spinach 4 oz shrimp (grilled/broiled) ¼ avocado	**Turkey Spinach Salad** Spinach 4 oz sliced deli turkey ¼ avocado	**Brussels Sprouts Medley & Chicken** Brussels sprouts, cauliflower, mushrooms (roasted) 4 oz chicken (roasted, skinless) 1 oz crumbled low-fat goat cheese
6 oz fat-free plain Greek yogurt 1 Tbsp pumpkin seeds	**Raspberry Smoothie** 1 cup almond milk 1 cup raspberries 2 tsp almond butter	6 oz fat-free plain Greek yogurt 1 Tbsp pumpkin seeds	**Raspberry Smoothie** 1 cup almond milk 1 cup raspberries 2 tsp almond butter
Shrimp Marinara 4 oz shrimp (steamed) ½ cup marinara sauce Burnt veggies (see page 197) 1 tsp capers 2 tsp olive oil	**Cod Cleanse** 4 oz cod (broiled) Broccoli (steamed) 2 tsp olive oil	**Vegetable & Chickpea Soup** Prepare 1 cup Tabatchnik vegetable soup per package and add ½ cup cooked chickpeas. Place in bowl and top with 3 Tbsp Parmesan cheese.	**Lemon Chicken & Artichoke** 4 oz chicken (marinated for up to 2 hours in 1 tsp minced garlic, 2 tsp olive oil, ½ cup lemon juice), grilled 1 small artichoke (steamed) and topped with 2 Tbsp fat-free plain Greek yogurt mixed with 2 tsp Dijon mustard

WEEK 3: Sip Your Way Slim

Keep a spritzer on your desk and use it to mist your face during the day.

Make a simple sage tea: Add boiling water to a teaspoon of chopped fresh sage and let it steep for 5 to 10 minutes before straining and drinking. Researchers say it will make you feel more alert and also calmer. (I like it with a little lime juice.)

BUY A PRETTY 1-LITER WATER BOTTLE AND LEAVE IT ON YOUR DESK AT WORK. IT WILL BE A DAILY REMINDER TO TANK UP.

Be a clock watcher: Some people find it helpful to set reminders on their phone or computer to take water breaks. I like to have a glass of water every time I have a snack.

Take tea with a twist: Try a tea you've never iced before, and make a small pitcher.

Freeze your water: If you like your water really cold, fill your water bottles, freeze them, and then toss them in your gym bag or work bag. They'll be melted but still frosty by the time you crack 'em open.

Having a cute little teapot may help encourage you to brew up a small pot of tea during the day or after dinner. Each mug of herbal tea helps hydrate you.

If your home is dry, add a humidifier. The additional moisture will help your breathing and your skin.

GO GREEN! TRY A GREEN JUICE, EVEN IF YOU DON'T THINK YOU CAN STOMACH IT. VEGETABLE JUICES ARE REFRESHING, HYDRATING, AND LIKE HAVING A SALAD IN A GLASS.

WEEK 4: Don't Get Stuck at the Gym

	Monday	Tuesday	Wednesday
Breakfast	**Energy Omelet** ½ cup cottage cheese and 2 oz deli turkey in omelet made with 1 whole egg plus 2 whites ⅓ cup cooked oatmeal	**Nutritious Life Power Bar** See page 173.	**Going Grainy** ⅓ cup cooked quinoa or oatmeal 1 hard-boiled egg Black pepper (to taste)
Snack 1	Sliced pear 2 oz part-skim ricotta ½ tsp cinnamon	¼ cup raisins 10 almonds	Sliced pear 2 oz part-skim ricotta ½ tsp cinnamon
Lunch	**Antipasto Platter** 2 Tbsp roasted red bell peppers 4 Tbsp hummus 1 oz low-fat feta cheese or 12 large olives 4 fiber crackers	**Turkey Salad** 2 cups chopped endive ½ cup cherry tomatoes 4 oz deli turkey 2 tsp olive oil Balsamic vinegar (to taste)	**Cheesy Chicken Melt** Romaine lettuce and tomato (for garnish) 4 oz chicken breast (grilled) 1 oz low-fat Cheddar cheese 1 slice Ezekiel bread
Snack 2	**Invigorate Shake** 1 cup low-fat milk ¼ avocado Juice of ½ lemon 1 tsp fresh mint	1 cup 1% Horizon organic chocolate milk 8 cashews	**Invigorate Shake** 1 cup low-fat milk ¼ avocado Juice of ½ lemon 1 tsp fresh mint
Dinner	**Tofu Kebabs & Spinach** 4 oz firm tofu, cubed and alternated on skewer with red and yellow peppers, red onions, mushrooms 1 cup spinach (steamed) 2 tsp toasted sesame oil	**Bison Un-Taco Salad** 4 oz bison sirloin steak (roasted) Romaine ¼ cup each chopped red bell peppers and tomatoes 2 Tbsp chopped red onion ⅓ cup kidney beans 1 Tbsp Monterey Jack cheese	**Burger to Bite** 4 oz 85% lean organic ground beef burger 1 oz Cheddar

Thursday	Friday	Saturday	Sunday
Keri's Favorite Smoothie 1 small banana 1 cup almond milk 1 tsp almond butter ⅛ avocado 1 cup ice	**Simple Scrambled Eggs** 1 whole egg plus 2 egg whites (scrambled) ½ tsp dried oregano	**Savory Quinoa** ⅓ cup cooked quinoa 2 oz part-skim ricotta cheese 3 Tbsp grated Parmesan cheese Black pepper (to taste)	**Mediterranean Scramble** 1 slice Ezekiel bread (toasted) 1 cup baby spinach 1 oz low-fat feta cheese 1 egg plus 2 whites 1 Tbsp chopped black olives
¼ cup raisins 10 almonds	Sliced pear 2 oz part-skim ricotta ½ tsp cinnamon	¼ cup raisins 10 almonds	Sliced pear 2 oz part-skim ricotta ½ tsp cinnamon
Asian Salad 1 cup chopped cabbage 4 oz tofu 8 chopped cashews 1 Tbsp rice vinegar 1 tsp Dijon mustard	**Salmon Spinach Salad** Spinach 4 oz salmon (broiled/grilled) ¼ avocado	**Crrrrunch Salad** 2 cups baby spinach 1 cup sliced cucumber 10 strips yellow bell pepper ½ cup chickpeas 18 pistachios 4 crumbled fiber crackers	**Tuna Tabbouleh** See page 178.
1 cup 1% Horizon organic chocolate milk 8 cashews	**Invigorate Shake** 1 cup low-fat milk ¼ avocado Juice of ½ lemon 1 tsp fresh mint	1 cup 1% Horizon organic chocolate milk 8 cashews	**Invigorate Shake** 1 cup low-fat milk ¼ avocado Juice of ½ lemon 1 tsp fresh mint
Pork Tenderloin & Bok Choy 4 oz pork tenderloin (grilled) Bok choy (steamed) 2 tsp olive oil	**Spicy Salsa Chicken** 4 oz chicken breast ½ cup salsa 2 tsp olive oil Balsamic vinegar (to taste) Asparagus (roasted)	**Scallops & Pea Puree** 4 oz broiled scallops ½ cup peas pureed with 2 tsp olive oil and ½ cup chopped basil	**Parmesan-Coated Halibut & Spicy Sprouts** See page 188.

WEEK 4: **Don't Get Stuck at the Gym**

In today's workout, think of one thing—just one!—that's outside your comfort zone and try it. That means running faster for a minute, lifting a slightly heavier weight, or pushing a 30-minute routine to 35.

Brush your teeth on one leg to challenge your balance.

UPDATE YOUR SPORTS GEAR, ESPECIALLY WORKOUT BRAS: DO THEY STILL OFFER PLENTY OF SUPPORT? DOES IT MAKE YOU FEEL GOOD TO WEAR THEM? NEW GEAR ALWAYS MOTIVATES ME.

Perfect your pushup. Whether you do them against the wall, from your knees, or full strength, take a second to check your posture— is your core strong?

Back it up: In a safe place, try walking backward. It challenges your coordination.

Tell yourself you can do it:
Sports psychologists learn more every day about how effective positive self-talk is, whether motivational ("I know I can finish this 5K because I've been training hard") or instructional ("Chin up, longer strides").

Sore? Exercise anyway. The newest research indicates that doing a low-intensity workout on your off days improves your ability to rebound.

Be a mighty mountain. This is one of the simplest yoga poses, but a great posture check: Stand so your big toes touch, and your heels are slightly apart, press your shoulders down, and hold arms overhead, palms facing each other. Imagine a string connected to the top of your head, straightening your spine.

Stock up on Epsom salts. Rich in magnesium, they can help soothe muscle soreness when you add them to a hot bath.

JUMP ROPE: CHEAP AND PORTABLE, JUMP ROPES CAN BE USED FOR A MEDIUM-INTENSITY WORKOUT, OR YOU CAN PICK UP THE PACE FOR MORE INTENSE INTERVALS.

WEEK 5: **Feel Sexy to Slim Down**

	Monday	Tuesday	Wednesday
Breakfast	**Awesome Avocado** 1 slice Ezekiel bread (toasted) 1/2 cup fat-free cottage cheese 1/4 avocado	**Going Grainy** 1/3 cup cooked quinoa or oatmeal 1 hard-boiled egg Black pepper (to taste)	**Energy Omelet** 1/2 cup cottage cheese and 2 oz deli turkey in omelet made with 1 whole egg plus 2 whites 1/3 cup cooked oatmeal
Snack 1	1/2 grapefruit 1/2 tsp cinnamon or ground cloves 1 Tbsp chopped pecans	1 cup cubed watermelon 15 crushed peanuts	1/2 grapefruit 1/2 tsp cinnamon or ground cloves 1 Tbsp chopped pecans
Lunch	**Vegetarian Chili** Add chopped bell pepper to 1 cup of Amy's organic vegetarian chili. Add 1 oz shredded Cheddar cheese.	**Tomato & Artichoke Shrimp** 1/2 cup cherry tomatoes 1/2 cup artichoke hearts 4 oz shrimp (steamed) 2 tsp olive oil Balsamic vinegar (to taste)	**Crrrrunch Salad** 2 cups baby spinach 1 cup sliced cucumber 10 strips yellow bell pepper 1/2 cup chickpeas 18 pistachios 4 crumbled fiber crackers
Snack 2	**Green Almond Butter Smoothie** 1 cup almond milk 1/2 tsp ground ginger 1 cup ice 2 tsp almond butter 3/4 cup spinach	6 oz fat-free plain Greek yogurt 1 Tbsp pumpkin seeds	**Green Almond Butter Smoothie** 1 cup almond milk 1/2 tsp ground ginger 1 cup ice 2 tsp almond butter 3/4 cup spinach
Dinner	**Jambalaya-Style Stir-Fry** See page 191.	**Cod Cleanse** 4 oz cod (broiled) 1/2 cup broccoli (steamed) 2 tsp olive oil	**Steak & Greens** 4 oz steak (grilled) Spinach (sautéed) Burnt veggies (See page 197.)

Thursday	Friday	Saturday	Sunday
Quinoa Crunch $\frac{1}{3}$ cup cooked quinoa 6 oz fat-free plain Greek yogurt 1 Tbsp chia seeds	**Simple Scrambled Eggs** 1 whole egg plus 2 egg whites (scrambled) $\frac{1}{2}$ tsp dried oregano	**Rise & Shine** 1 cup mango chunks 6 oz fat-free plain Greek yogurt 1 Tbsp sunflower seeds	**Coconut Quinoa Pudding** $\frac{1}{3}$ cup cooked quinoa 6 oz fat-free plain Greek yogurt 2 Tbsp grated fresh coconut
1 cup cubed watermelon 15 crushed peanuts	$\frac{1}{2}$ grapefruit $\frac{1}{2}$ tsp cinnamon or ground cloves 1 Tbsp chopped pecans	1 cup cubed watermelon 15 crushed peanuts	$\frac{1}{2}$ grapefruit $\frac{1}{2}$ tsp cinnamon or ground cloves 1 Tbsp chopped pecans
Easy Egg Salad 2 cups chopped romaine 2 hard-boiled eggs 2 Tbsp fat-free plain Greek yogurt 1 Tbsp Dijon mustard 1 tsp olive oil	**Salmon Salad Wrap** 4 lettuce leaves, as wraps 10 strips red bell pepper $\frac{1}{4}$ cup diced red onion 2 tsp capers 4 oz salmon (grilled) 2 tsp fat-free plain yogurt 2 tsp olive oil	**Cheesy Chicken Melt** Romaine lettuce and tomato (for garnish) 4 oz chicken breast (grilled) 1 oz low-fat Cheddar cheese 1 slice Ezekiel bread	**Greek Salad** 2 cups chopped romaine $\frac{1}{2}$ cup sliced cucumber $\frac{1}{4}$ cup artichoke hearts $\frac{1}{2}$ cup sliced tomato $\frac{1}{2}$ cup cooked lentils 2 oz low-fat feta cheese
6 oz fat-free plain Greek yogurt 1 Tbsp pumpkin seeds	**Green Almond Butter Smoothie** 1 cup almond milk $\frac{1}{2}$ tsp ground ginger 1 cup ice 2 tsp almond butter $\frac{3}{4}$ cup spinach	6 oz fat-free plain Greek yogurt 1 Tbsp pumpkin seeds	**Green Almond Butter Smoothie** 1 cup almond milk $\frac{1}{2}$ tsp ground ginger 1 cup ice 2 tsp almond butter $\frac{3}{4}$ cup spinach
Shrimp Marinara 4 oz shrimp (steamed) $\frac{1}{2}$ cup marinara sauce Burnt veggies (See page 197.) 1 tsp capers 2 tsp olive oil	**Tofu Kebabs & Spinach** 4 oz firm tofu, cubed and skewered with red and yellow peppers, red onions, mushrooms 1 cup spinach (steamed) 2 tsp toasted sesame oil	**Lemon Chicken & Artichoke** 4 oz chicken (marinated for up to 2 hours in 1 tsp minced garlic, 2 tsp olive oil, $\frac{1}{2}$ cup lemon juice), grilled 1 small artichoke (steamed) and topped with 2 Tbsp fat-free plain Greek yogurt mixed with 2 tsp Dijon mustard	**Lentil Spinach Salad with Salmon** Spinach $\frac{1}{2}$ cup cooked lentils 4 oz salmon (grilled/ broiled) 2 tsp olive oil

WEEK 5: **Feel Sexy to Slim Down**

Try a libido-boosting yoga move:
The wide-legged straddle pose,
where you simply sit down, open your legs
in as wide a V as is comfortable,
then lower your head and chest toward
the floor, increases blood flow in
the pelvic region.

Buy a better bathrobe. A spa-worthy robe will remind you that, yes, you, you domestic goddess, should spend more time lounging around the house! Few things feel as sexy as a silk kimono.

Invest in electric candles.
Real candles can be great for romantic
atmosphere and aromatherapy,
but LED candles set the mood and alleviate
any worries. (Who wants to be distracted
from sex or sleep by thinking,
"Wait, did I blow out the candles?")

Add vanilla to your
flavor repertoire.
A little vanilla extract
(besides smelling like heaven)
may relieve anxiety,
perk up your libido,
and help wrangle
free radicals.

FIND YOURSELF A SEXY ACTION-HERO
ROLE MODEL. MAYBE IT'S GINA CARANO
IN *HAYWIRE*, MRS. PEEL FROM
THE AVENGERS, OR EVEN WONDER
WOMAN. (I STILL LOVE ANGELINA JOLIE
AS LARA CROFT.) POST A PICTURE
SOMEWHERE YOU CAN SEE IT.

If you have not been
doing your 8-count
breath daily—do it!
You will be surprised
at how lowering stress
can lead to sexiness!

Eat More, Not Less + Breathe Your Way Thin + Sip Your Way Slim + Don't Get Stuck at the Gym + **Feel Sexy to Slim Down** + Put Yourself First + Always Sleep Alone + Clean Out Your Closet

WEEK 6: **Put Yourself First**

	Monday	Tuesday	Wednesday
Breakfast	**Energy Waffle** 1 whole grain waffle 1 cup rice milk 2 tsp peanut butter	**Spiced Fig & Ricotta Toast** See page 172.	**Awesome Avocado** 1 slice Ezekiel bread (toasted) 1/2 cup fat-free cottage cheese 1/4 avocado
Snack 1	2 tsp coconut butter 1 fiber cracker Cucumber slices	1 small orange 4 Brazil nuts	2 tsp coconut butter 1 fiber-rich cracker Cucumber slices
Lunch	**Turkey Salad** 2 cups chopped endive 1/2 cup cherry tomatoes 4 oz sliced deli turkey 2 tsp olive oil Balsamic vinegar (to taste)	**Slim Slaw with Shrimp** 1/2 cup sliced red cabbage 1/2 cup sliced green cabbage 4 oz grilled shrimp 1/4 cup sliced almonds 1 Tbsp rice vinegar 1 tsp Dijon mustard	**Salmon Salad Wrap** 4 lettuce leaves, as wraps 10 strips red bell pepper 1/4 cup diced red onion 2 tsp capers 4 oz salmon (grilled) 2 tsp fat-free plain yogurt 2 tsp olive oil
Snack 2	6 oz plain fat-free Greek yogurt Fresh coconut shavings 1/2 tsp cinnamon	Papaya with lime juice 1 oz low-fat mozzarella cheese	6 oz plain fat-free Greek yogurt Fresh coconut shavings 1/2 tsp cinnamon
Dinner	**Lentil Spinach Salad & Chicken** 4 oz chicken (grilled/broiled) Spinach 1/2 cup cooked lentils 2 tsp olive oil	**Easy Chili** 4 oz cooked ground turkey 1/4 cup bell pepper 1/4 cup tomato sauce 1/4 cup pinto beans 2 tsp olive oil 1 oz Cheddar cheese	**Pork Tenderlion & Bok Choy** 4 oz pork tenderloin (grilled) 2 tsp olive oil Bok choy (steamed)

Thursday	Friday	Saturday	Sunday
Coconut Quinoa Pudding ⅓ cup cooked quinoa 6 oz fat-free plain Greek yogurt 2 Tbsp grated fresh coconut	**Savory Oatmeal** ⅓ cup cooked oatmeal 2 oz part-skim ricotta cheese 3 tsp grated Parmesan cheese Black pepper (to taste)	**Mediterranean Scramble** 1 slice Ezekiel bread (toasted) 1 cup baby spinach 1 oz low-fat feta cheese 1 egg plus 2 whites 1 Tbsp chopped black olives	**Peanut Butter Cup Oatmeal** See page 167.
1 small orange 4 Brazil nuts	2 tsp coconut butter 1 fiber cracker Cucumber slices	1 small orange 4 Brazil nuts	2 tsp coconut butter 1 fiber cracker Cucumber slices
Salmon Spinach Salad Spinach 4 oz salmon (grilled/broiled) ¼ avocado	**Greek Salad** 2 cups chopped romaine ½ cup sliced cucumber ¼ cup artichoke hearts ½ cup sliced tomato ½ cup cooked lentils 2 oz reduced-fat feta cheese	**Asian Salad** 1 cup chopped cabbage 4 oz tofu 8 chopped cashews 1 Tbsp rice vinegar 1 tsp Dijon mustard	**Cheesy Chicken Melt** 4 oz chicken breast (grilled) 1 oz low-fat Cheddar cheese 1 slice Ezekiel bread Romaine lettuce and tomato (for garnish)
Papaya with lime juice 1 oz low-fat mozzarella cheese	6 oz plain fat-free Greek yogurt Fresh coconut shavings ½ tsp cinnamon	Papaya with lime juice 1 oz low-fat mozzarella cheese	6 oz plain fat-free Greek yogurt Fresh coconut shavings ½ tsp cinnamon
Bison Un-Taco Salad 4 oz bison sirloin steak (roasted) Romaine ¼ cup each chopped red bell peppers and tomatoes 2 Tbsp chopped red onion ⅓ cup kidney beans 1 Tbsp Monterey Jack cheese	**Scallops & Pea Puree** 4 oz scallops ½ cup peas pureed with 2 tsp olive oil and ½ cup chopped basil	**Spicy Salsa Chicken** 4 oz chicken breast ½ cup salsa 2 tsp olive oil Balsamic vinegar (to taste) Asparagus (roasted)	**Lentil Spinach Salad & Salmon** 4 oz salmon (grilled/broiled) Spinach ½ cup cooked lentils 2 tsp olive oil

WEEK 6: **Put Yourself First**

Have a "redefining beauty" breakthrough:
What are your three favorite nonphysical traits about yourself and others?

Give yourself a scalp massage. I use about a half cup of my best olive oil with a few drops of essential oil (rosemary is one of my faves, as is bergamot) and rub it into my scalp with tiny circular motions. Wait 10 minutes, and then shampoo— your hair will look great, and you'll feel incredible.

FUN WITH YOUR FEET:
WHEN YOU DON'T HAVE THE TIME
OR ENERGY FOR THE WHOLE
HOT-BATH ROUTINE,
JUST PUT ENOUGH WATER
IN THE TUB TO COVER YOUR
FEET AND ADD A
FAVORITE ESSENTIAL OIL.

Eat More, Not Less + Breathe Your Way Thin + Sip Your Way Slim + Don't Get Stuck at the Gym + Feel Sexy to Slim Down + **Put Yourself First** + Always Sleep Alone + Clean Out Your Closet

Coddle your cuticles.
No one likes hangnails,
and I find it soothing to
massage my cuticles with
my own mixture of
olive oil and almond oil.

Skip a shampoo.
Experts say hair looks its best
when its natural oils are
allowed to reach the ends,
and that can take a day or two.
Use that extra 15 minutes
to sip your morning
coffee, not chug it!

Go the gym—*not*.
Take a trip to the gym
or the local Y,
but skip the machines
and classes and
head straight
to the steam room
or sauna.

WEEK 7: Always Sleep Alone

	Monday	Tuesday	Wednesday
Breakfast	**Coconut Quinoa Pudding** ⅓ cup cooked quinoa 6 oz fat-free plain Greek yogurt 2 Tbsp grated fresh coconut	**Refreshing Grapefruit** ½ grapefruit 6 oz fat-free plain yogurt 1 hard-boiled egg	**Peanut Butter Cup Oatmeal** See page 169.
Snack 1	Celery 2 Tbsp hummus	2 dried apricots 8 pecan halves	Celery 2 Tbsp hummus
Lunch	**Cheesy Chicken Melt** 4 oz chicken breast (grilled) 1 oz low-fat Cheddar cheese 1 slice Ezekiel bread Romaine lettuce and tomato (for garnish)	**Chicken Spinach Salad** Spinach 4 oz chicken (grilled/broiled) ¼ avocado	**Vegetable & Chickpea Soup** Prepare 1 cup Tabatchnik vegetable soup per package and add ½ cup cooked chickpeas. Place in bowl and top with 3 Tbsp Parmesan cheese.
Snack 2	½ cup cottage cheese ½ cup pineapple chunks	**Chamomile Tea Latte** 2 oz steamed low-fat milk Chamomile tea ¼ tsp nutmeg	½ cup cottage cheese ½ cup pineapple chunks
Dinner	**Parmesan-Coated Halibut & Spicy Sprouts** See page 188.	**Shrimp Marinara** 4 oz shrimp (steamed) ½ cup marinara sauce Burnt veggies (see page 197.) 1 tsp capers 2 tsp olive oil	**Tofu Kebabs & Spinach** 4 oz firm tofu, cubed and alternated on skewer with red and yellow peppers, red onions, mushrooms Spinach (steamed)

Thursday	Friday	Saturday	Sunday
Keri's Favorite Smoothie 1 small banana 1 cup almond milk 1 tsp almond butter ⅛ avocado 1 cup ice	**Energy Omelet** ⅓ cup cooked oatmeal ½ cup cottage cheese 1 whole egg plus 2 whites 2 oz deli turkey	**Mediterranean Scramble** 1 slice Ezekiel bread (toasted) 1 cup baby spinach 1 oz low-fat feta cheese 1 egg plus 2 whites 1 Tbsp chopped black olives	**Caprese Breakfast** 1 slice Ezekiel bread (toasted) 3 oz low-fat mozzarella cheese 2 tsp olive oil 1 slice tomato
2 dried apricots 8 pecan halves	Celery 2 Tbsp hummus	2 dried apricots 8 pecan halves	Celery 2 Tbsp hummus
Tuna Tabbouleh See page 178.	**Mini Roasted Veggie Wraps** 10 strips red bell pepper ¼ cup grilled zucchini ¼ cup grilled eggplant 3 oz low-fat feta cheese 2 tsp olive oil 2 small corn tortillas	**Tomato & Artichoke Shrimp** ½ cup cherry tomatoes ½ cup artichoke hearts 4 oz cooked shrimp 2 tsp olive oil Balsamic vinegar (to taste)	**Antipasto Platter** 2 Tbsp roasted red bell peppers 4 Tbsp hummus 4 fiber crackers 1 oz low-fat feta cheese *or* 12 large olives
Chamomile Tea Latte 2 oz steamed low-fat milk Chamomile tea ¼ tsp nutmeg 8 almonds	½ cup cottage cheese ½ cup pineapple chunks	½ cup cottage cheese ½ cup pineapple chunks	**Chamomile Tea Latte** 2 oz steamed low-fat milk Chamomile tea ¼ tsp nutmeg 8 almonds
Lentil Spinach Salad & Shrimp Spinach ½ cup cooked lentils 4 oz shrimp (grilled) 2 tsp olive oil	**Steak & Sautéed Spinach** 4 oz steak (grilled) Spinach (sautéed) 2 tsp olive oil	**Lemon Chicken & Artichoke** 4 oz chicken (marinated for up to 2 hours in 1 tsp minced garlic, 2 tsp olive oil, ½ cup lemon juice), grilled 1 small artichoke (steamed) and topped with 2 Tbsp fat-free plain Greek yogurt mixed with 2 tsp Dijon mustard	**Bison Un-Taco Salad** 4 oz bison sirloin steak (roasted) Romaine ¼ cup each chopped red bell peppers and tomatoes 2 Tbsp chopped red onion ⅓ cup kidney beans 1 Tbsp Monterey Jack cheese

WEEK 7: **Always Sleep Alone**

Check the temperature in the bedroom: 66°F is optimal.

Borrow a white noise machine for a test-drive. (Don't buy one until you do—they annoy some people.)

TURN YOUR MATTRESS, AND WHILE YOU'RE AT IT, TRY TO REMEMBER WHEN YOU BOUGHT IT: MANY PEOPLE SLEEP BETTER AFTER THEY REPLACE AN 8- TO 10-YEAR-OLD MATTRESS.

Put a notepad by your bed so you can jot down dreams: They help us work through unresolved emotions and give us information about our health.

Try to even out your schedule so you can turn in at the same time each night, even on weekends.

Rethink your blankets. Weighted blankets are used in psychiatric hospitals to calm patients, and while that may be a little extreme, you get the idea: Heavy blankets feel like a warm hug. Experiment with different weights.

Time yourself. It should take no more than 30 minutes to fall asleep each night. If it takes longer, it's time to change up your routine.

Switch to lower-wattage bulbs in the bedroom to make it more soothing.

SEND WORRIES UP TO THE SKY: VISUALIZE THE THINGS THAT ARE BOTHERING YOU AS BALLOONS, WHICH YOU CAN RELEASE. (SOME PEOPLE SAY IMAGINING THEMSELVES ACTUALLY PUTTING WORRIES ON A SHELF WORKS BETTER.)

Don't use your iPad for bedtime reading. Some experts suspect backlit devices can interfere with melatonin levels.

Reward yourself for improving your sleep routine! Why not—you give yourself incentives for weight loss, right? Treat yourself to a pretty new sheet set or an aromatherapy alarm clock.

WEEK 8: Clean Out Your Closet

	Monday	Tuesday	Wednesday
Breakfast	**Energy Omelet** 1/3 cup cooked oatmeal 1/2 cup cottage cheese 1 whole egg plus 2 whites 2 oz deli turkey	**Savory Oatmeal** 1/3 cup cooked oatmeal 2 oz ricotta cheese 3 tsp grated Parmesan cheese 1/2 tsp black pepper	**Refreshing Grapefruit** 1/2 grapefruit 6 oz fat-free plain yogurt 1 hard-boiled egg
Snack 1	Red peppers 8 pecans halves	1 whole endive 8 cashews	Red peppers 8 pecans halves
Lunch	**Lentil Salad** 2 cups arugula 1/2 cup cooked lentils 1/2 cup cherry tomatoes 1/4 cup diced red onion 2 tsp olive oil	**Turkey Salad** 2 cups chopped endive 1/2 cup cherry tomatoes 4 oz sliced deli turkey 2 tsp olive oil Balsamic vinegar (to taste)	**Greek Salad** 2 cups chopped romaine 1/2 cup sliced cucumber 1/4 cup artichoke hearts 1/2 cup sliced tomato 1/2 cup cooked lentils 2 oz reduced-fat feta cheese
Snack 2	6 oz plain fat-free Greek yogurt 18 pistachios 1 tsp honey	6 oz plain fat-free Greek yogurt 2 tsp peanut butter 1/2 tsp cinnamon	6 oz plain fat-free Greek yogurt 18 pistachios 1 tsp honey
Dinner	**Lentil Spinach Salad with Chicken** 4 oz chicken (grilled/broiled) Spinach 1/2 cup cooked lentils 2 tsp olive oil	**Bison Un-Taco Salad** 4 oz bison sirloin steak (roasted) Romaine 1/4 cup each chopped red bell peppers and tomatoes 2 Tbsp chopped red onion 1/3 cup kidney beans 1 Tbsp Monterey Jack cheese	**Jambalaya-Style Stir-Fry** See page 191.

Thursday	Friday	Saturday	Sunday
Rise & Shine 1 cup mango chunks 6 oz fat-free plain Greek yogurt 1 Tbsp sunflower seeds	**Awesome Avocado** 1 slice Ezekiel bread (toasted) ½ cup fat-free cottage cheese ¼ avocado	**Coconut Quinoa Pudding** ⅓ cup cooked quinoa 6 oz fat-free plain Greek yogurt 2 Tbsp grated fresh coconut	**Spiced Fig & Ricotta Toast** See page 172.
1 whole endive 8 cashews	Red peppers 8 pecans halves	1 whole endive 8 cashews	Red peppers 8 pecans halves
Asian Salad 1 cup chopped cabbage 4 oz tofu 8 chopped cashews 1 Tbsp rice vinegar 1 tsp Dijon mustard	**Salmon Salad Wrap** 4 lettuce leaves, as wraps 10 strips red bell pepper ¼ cup diced red onion 2 tsp capers 4 oz salmon (grilled) 2 tsp fat-free plain yogurt 2 tsp olive oil	**Tomato & Artichoke Shrimp** ½ cup cherry tomatoes ½ cup artichoke hearts 4 oz cooked shrimp 2 tsp olive oil Balsamic vinegar (to taste)	**Vegetarian Chili** ¼ cup bell pepper ¼ cup tomato sauce ¼ cup pinto beans ¼ cup black beans
6 oz plain fat-free Greek yogurt 2 tsp peanut butter ½ tsp cinnamon	6 oz plain fat-free Greek yogurt 18 pistachios 1 tsp honey	6 oz plain fat-free Greek yogurt 2 tsp peanut butter ½ tsp cinnamon	6 oz plain fat-free Greek yogurt 18 pistachios 1 tsp honey
Pork Tenderloin & Bok Choy 4 oz pork tenderloin (grilled) 2 tsp olive oil Bok choy (steamed)	**Lemon Chicken & Artichoke** 4 oz chicken (marinated for up to 2 hours in 1 tsp minced garlic, 2 tsp olive oil, ½ cup lemon juice), grilled 1 small artichoke (steamed) and topped with 2 Tbsp fat-free plain Greek yogurt mixed with 2 tsp Dijon mustard	**Parmesan-Coated Halibut & Spicy Sprouts** See page 188.	**Scallops & Pea Puree** 4 oz scallops ½ cup peas pureed with 2 tsp olive oil and ½ cup chopped basil

WEEK 8: **Clean Out Your Closet**

Take 5 minutes to eliminate
germs and chemicals on your
kitchen counters:
Mix 1 gallon of warm water
with 1 cup of vinegar
(add a few drops of essential oil
if you don't like the smell)
and wipe down counters,
cupboards, and appliances.
Then, peek under the sink
at all your cleaners and get rid
three that you don't use—
the fewer chemicals
in your home, the better.

Simplify your recycling
system, in a way that makes
it easy to rinse cans and bottles
before tossing them in the bin.
(That way, they won't smell
or attract bugs.)

CONQUER CLUTTER. NEXT TIME YOU'RE IN
YOUR BATHROOM OR KITCHEN, LOOK
AROUND, GRAB THREE SELDOM-USED
THINGS, AND STASH 'EM IN A DRAWER.

Make a conscious effort to cut down on the food you end up throwing out: Food waste is the biggest component of landfills, and it's bad for your budget and the planet, since it produces damaging methane gas. If you don't do it already, start with a simple form of composting.

Organize your desk area. You will be more productive and may just have more time to go to the gym.

ORGANIZE THE FRIDGE. CUT, CHOP, AND PLACE VEGGIES IN GLASS CONTAINERS. MAKE IT LOOK PRETTY. I PROMISE, YOU WILL WANT TO EAT HEALTHIER WHEN YOU OPEN THE DOOR.

Eat More, Not Less + Breathe Your Way Thin + Sip Your Way Slim + Don't Get Stuck at the Gym + Feel Sexy to Slim Down + Put Yourself First + Always Sleep Alone + Clean Out Your Closet

Grocery Lists

Week 1

Produce

FRESH FRUIT
7 Granny Smith apples
2 avocados
3 lemons or 1 package
 of lemon juice

FRESH VEGETABLES
Spinach
Broccoli
Bok choy

Eggs

19 DHA-fortified eggs

Nuts, Butters, Seeds

6 tsp peanut butter

Oils

Cold-pressed olive oil

Grocery

GRAINS
1 cup quinoa
1 cup oatmeal

**OTHER
PACKAGED FOODS**
2 cups lentils
3½ cups artichoke
 hearts

Poultry

8 oz chicken
4 oz sliced deli turkey

Seafood

4 oz shrimp
4 oz cod
16 oz salmon

Meats

4 oz pork tenderloin

Herbs & Spices

Dried oregano
Black pepper
Cinnamon

Week 2

Produce

FRESH FRUIT
1 banana
1 avocado
1 lemon

FRESH VEGETABLES
1 tomato
$\frac{1}{2}$ cup cherry tomatoes
1 package carrots
Spinach
1 small cucumber
1 yellow bell pepper
Arugula
Celery
$\frac{1}{4}$ cup diced red onion
2 red bell peppers
1 zucchini
1 small eggplant
Broccoli
Cauliflower
Bok choy
1 cup brussels sprouts

Dairy

30 oz fat-free plain Greek yogurt
3 cups almond milk
2 oz part-skim ricotta cheese
5 Tbsp grated Parmesan cheese
1 oz low-fat mozzarella cheese
4 oz low-fat feta cheese
2 cups soy milk
1 oz Cheddar cheese

Eggs

7 DH-fortified eggs

Nuts, Butters, Seeds

1 Tbsp chia seeds
56 cashews
18 pistachios
8 Tbsp flaxseed
1 tsp almond butter

Oils

Cold-pressed olive oil

Grocery

GRAINS
$\frac{2}{3}$ cup quinoa
$\frac{1}{3}$ cup oatmeal

BREADS, CRACKERS
1 slice Ezekiel bread
8 fiber crackers
2 corn tortillas

OTHER PACKAGED FOODS
$\frac{1}{2}$ cup marinara sauce
3 green tea bags
1 tsp capers
$\frac{1}{2}$ cup chickpeas
$\frac{1}{2}$ cup lentils
4 Tbsp hummus

Poultry

8 oz chicken

Seafood

8 oz salmon
4 oz shrimp
4 oz cod
4 oz halibut

Meats

4 oz 85% organic ground beef burger
4 oz pork tenderloin
4 oz steak

Herbs & Spices

Black pepper
Dried oregano
Chili pepper flakes

Week 3

Produce

FRESH FRUIT
2 avocados
3 cups fresh raspberries
3 cups frozen
 raspberries
2 lemons
1 banana

FRESH VEGETABLES
Kale
Celery
Romaine lettuce
5 cucumbers
2 cups chopped endive
1/2 cup cherry tomatoes
1 red pepper
2 yellow bell pepper
1 red cabbage
1 green cabbage
Brussels sprouts
Cauliflower
Mushrooms
Bok choy
Baby spinach
1 onion
1 head broccoli
1 artichoke

Dairy

30 oz fat-free Greek
 yogurt, plus 2 Tbsp
5 cups almond milk
1/2 cup fat-free cottage
 cheese
4 oz low-fat goat cheese
3 Tbsp grated Parmesan
 cheese

Eggs

7 DHA-fortified eggs

Nuts, Butters, Seeds

1 Tbsp chia seeds
9 tsp almond butter
50 almonds
18 pistachios
3 Tbsp pumpkin seeds

Oils

Cold-pressed olive oil
2 tsp toasted sesame oil

Grocery

GRAINS
2/3 cup quinoa
1/3 cup oatmeal

BREADS, CRACKERS
1 slice Ezekiel bread
4 fiber crackers

**OTHER PACKAGED
FOODS**
1 cup chickpeas
1/2 cup lentils
1 tsp capers
1/2 cup marinara sauce
1 tsp minced garlic
Minced ginger
1/2 tsp matcha green tea
 powder
1 cup Tabatchnik
 vegetable soup

Poultry

8 oz deli turkey
12 oz chicken

Seafood

4 oz salmon
12 oz shrimp
4 oz cod

Meats

4 oz pork tenderloin

Vegetarian

4 oz tofu

Herbs & Spices

Black pepper
Dried oregano

Condiments

Dijon mustard
Rice wine vinegar
Balsamic vinegar

Week 4

Produce

FRESH FRUIT
4 avocados
1 banana
4 pears
2 lemons

FRESH VEGETABLES
Baby spinach
1 red bell pepper
2 cups chopped endive
$\frac{1}{2}$ cup cherry tomatoes
Romaine lettuce
1 cup cabbage
$\frac{1}{4}$ cup grape tomatoes
Brussels sprouts
Asparagus
2 cucumbers
2 yellow bell peppers
2 red bell peppers
2 red onions
Mushrooms
1 small sweet potato
Bok choy
$\frac{1}{2}$ cup peas
1 tomato

Dairy

3 oz low-fat feta cheese
6 Tbsp grated Parmesan cheese
8 oz part-skim ricotta cheese
2 oz low-fat Cheddar cheese
4 cups low-fat milk
3 cups 1% Horizon organic chocolate milk
1 Tbsp Monterey Jack cheese
1 cup almond milk
$\frac{1}{2}$ cup cottage cheese

Eggs

10 DHA-fortified eggs

Nuts, Butters, Seeds

30 almonds
1 tsp almond butter
32 cashews
18 pistachios
$\frac{1}{4}$ cup ground flaxseed
$\frac{1}{2}$ cup cashew or almond butter

Oils

Cold-pressed olive oil
2 tsp toasted sesame oil

Grocery

GRAINS
$\frac{2}{3}$ cup quinoa
1 cup oatmeal

BREADS, CRACKERS
8 fiber crackers
2 slices Ezekiel bread

OTHER PACKAGED FOODS
1 box raisins
4 Tbsp hummus
$\frac{1}{2}$ cup chickpeas
$\frac{1}{3}$ cup kidney beans
$\frac{1}{2}$ cup dried apricots
$\frac{1}{4}$ cup honey
$\frac{1}{4}$ cup unsweetened dried cranberries or goji berries
$\frac{1}{4}$ cup shredded unsweetened coconut
12 large olives
$\frac{1}{4}$ cup salsa

Poultry

6 oz deli turkey
8 oz chicken

Seafood

4 oz salmon
4 oz scallops
4 oz halibut
5 oz chunk light tuna in
 water

Meats

4 oz bison sirloin steak
4 oz 85% lean organic
 ground beef
4 oz pork tenderloin

Vegetarian

8 oz tofu

Herbs & Spices

Parsley
Mint
Basil
Ground cinnamon
Ground nutmeg
Ground ginger
Chili pepper flakes
Dried oregano
Black pepper
Sea salt

Condiments

Dijon mustard
Rice wine vinegar
Balsamic vinegar
Red wine vinegar

Week 5

Produce

FRESH FRUIT
1 avocado
1 mango
2 Tbsp fresh grated coconut
2 grapefruits
1 watermelon
2 lemons

FRESH VEGETABLES
Baby spinach
4 large lettuce leaves
Romaine lettuce
2 tomatoes
1/2 cup cherry tomatoes
1 cucumber
2 yellow bell peppers
2 red bell peppers
Broccoli
2 red onions
Mushrooms
1/2 cup artichoke hearts
1 small artichoke
Celery
Green bell pepper

Dairy

36 oz fat-free plain Greek yogurt, plus 4 Tbsp
2 oz low-fat Cheddar cheese
4 cups almond milk
1 cup fat-free cottage cheese
2 oz low-fat feta cheese

Eggs

9 DHA-fortified eggs

Nuts, Butters, Seeds

3 Tbsp pumpkin seeds
8 tsp almond butter
8 cashews
45 peanuts
4 Tbsp chopped pecans
1 Tbsp chia seeds
1 Tbsp sunflower seeds
18 pistachios

Oils

Cold-pressed olive oil
2 tsp toasted sesame oil

Grocery

GRAINS
1 cup quinoa
2/3 cup oatmeal
1/3 cup black or brown rice

BREADS
2 slices Ezekiel bread
4 fiber crackers

OTHER PACKAGED FOODS
1/4 cup tomato sauce
1/4 cup black beans
1/4 cup pinto beans
1/2 cup chickpeas
3 tsp capers
1/2 cup marinara sauce
2 tsp minced garlic
1 cup lentils
1 cup Amy's organic vegetarian chili

Poultry

8 oz chicken
2 oz deli turkey

Seafood

8 oz salmon
4 oz cod
8 oz shrimp
3 oz wild rock or small
 shrimp

Meats

4 oz steak

Vegetarian

4 oz tofu

Herbs & Spices

Parsley
Dried oregano
Ground cloves
Ground ginger
Ground red pepper
Black pepper

Condiments

Dijon mustard
Balsamic vinegar

Week 6

Produce

FRESH FRUIT
1 avocado
3 papayas
3 oranges
1 lime or lime juice
1 Black Mission fig

FRESH VEGETABLES
Spinach
1 green cabbage
1 red cabbage
Bok choy
Romaine lettuce
2 cups chopped endive
2 cucumbers
1 yellow bell pepper
2 red bell peppers
2 red onions
3 tomatoes
1/2 cup cherry tomatoes
1/2 cup peas
Asparagus

Dairy

25 oz fat-free plain Greek yogurt, plus 2 tsp
1 cup rice milk
2 oz part-skim ricotta cheese
1/2 cup fat-free cottage cheese
3 tsp Parmesan cheese
3 oz reduced-fat feta cheese
3 oz low-fat mozzarella cheese
1 Tbsp Monterey jack cheese
2 oz low-fat Cheddar cheese

Eggs

3 DHA-fortified eggs

Nuts, Butters, Seeds

2 Tbsp peanut butter
8 tsp coconut butter
12 Brazil nuts
1/4 cup sliced almonds
8 chopped cashews
1 Tbsp chopped walnuts
2 tsp smooth peanut butter

Oils

Cold-pressed olive oil

Grocery

GRAINS
1/3 cup quinoa
1/3 cup cooked oatmeal
1/2 cup old-fashioned rolled oats

BREADS
4 slices Ezekiel bread
1 whole-grain waffle
1 Thomas' Light Multi-Grain English Muffin
4 fiber crackers

OTHER PACKAGED FOODS
1/4 cup artichoke hearts
1/3 cup kidney beans
1/4 cup pinto beans
1/4 cup tomato sauce
1/2 cup salsa
1 1/2 cup lentils
Black olives
1 tsp maple syrup or honey
1/4 tsp minced ginger
2 tsp dark chocolate chips
2 tsp fresh grated coconut

Poultry

12 oz chicken
4 oz ground turkey
4 oz sliced deli turkey

Seafood

12 oz salmon
4 oz scallops
4 oz shrimp

Meats

4 oz pork tenderloin
4 oz bison sirloin steak

Vegetarian

4 oz tofu

Herbs & Spices

Fresh basil
Ground cinnamon
Ground nutmeg
Black pepper

Condiments

Rice wine vinegar
Dijon mustard
Balsamic vinegar

Week 7

Produce

FRESH FRUIT
1 small banana
1 grapefruit
1 avocado
1 pineapple
2 lemons

FRESH VEGETABLES
Spinach
1 stalk celery
½ cup cherry tomatoes
2 tomatoes
Romaine lettuce
2 red bell peppers
2 yellow bell peppers
Broccoli
2 red onions
1 zucchini
1 eggplant
½ cup artichoke hearts
Mushrooms
1 small artichoke
1 cucumber
Brussels sprouts

Dairy

12 oz fat-free plain Greek yogurt, plus 2 Tbsp
1 cup almond milk
3 oz low-fat mozzarella cheese
2½ cups fat-free cottage cheese
2 oz low-fat Cheddar cheese
4 oz low-fat feta cheese
2½ cups fat-free milk
1 Tbsp Monterey Jack cheese
3 Tbsp grated Parmesean cheese

Eggs

7 DHA-fortified eggs

Nuts, Butters, Seeds

1 tsp almond butter
12 pecans
2 tsp smooth peanut butter

Oils

Cold-pressed olive oil

Grocery

GRAINS
⅔ cup quinoa
1 cup oatmeal

BREADS
2 small corn tortillas
1 whole-wheat pita
2 slices Ezekiel bread
4 fiber crackers

OTHER PACKAGED FOODS
16 Tbsp hummus
2 Tbsp roasted bell peppers
3 chamomile tea bags
12 large olives
1 tsp capers
½ cup marinara sauce
½ cup lentils
1 tsp minced garlic
⅓ cup kidney beans
1 tsp honey
¼ tsp unsweetened cocoa powder
2 tsp dark chocolate chips
6 dried apricots
2 Tbsp fresh grated coconut

Poultry

12 oz chicken
2 oz deli turkey

Seafood

4 oz skinless wild halibut
4 oz cod
12 oz shrimp
5 oz can chunk light
 tuna packed in water

Meats

4 oz steak
4 oz bison sirloin steak

Vegetarian

4 oz tofu

Herbs & Spices

Parsley
Dried oregano
Chili pepper flakes
Ground nutmeg

Condiments

Balsamic vinegar
Red wine vinegar

Week 8

Produce

FRESH FRUIT
1 avocado
1 mango
1 grapefruit
1 lemon
1 Black Mission fig

FRESH VEGETABLES
Baby spinach
Arugula
Romaine lettuce
1 tomato
1½ cups cherry
 tomatoes
1 cucumber
2 yellow bell peppers
4 red bell peppers
4 red onions
Bok choy
1 cabbage
1 cup artichoke hearts
4 heads endive
1 small artichoke
1 stalk celery
1 cup brussels sprouts
½ cup peas
Green bell pepper

Dairy

60 oz fat-free plain
 Greek yogurt, plus
 4 Tbsp
6 tsp grated Parmesan
 cheese
2 Tbsp grated Pecorino
1 cup fat-free cottage
 cheese
2 oz reduced-fat feta
 cheese
1 Tbsp Monterey Jack
 cheese
4 oz part-skim ricotta
 cheese

Eggs

4 DHA-fortified eggs

Nuts, Butters, Seeds

32 pecan halves
32 cashews
72 pistachios
6 tsp peanut butter
1 Tbsp sunflower seeds
1 Tbsp chopped walnuts

Oils

Cold-pressed olive oil

Grocery

GRAINS
1 cup quinoa
⅔ cup oatmeal
⅓ cup black or brown
 rice

BREAD
1 slice Ezekiel bread
1 Thomas' Light
 Multi-Grain English
 Muffin

**OTHER PACKAGED
FOODS**
¼ cup black beans
¼ cup pinto beans
⅓ cup kidney beans
1½ cups lentils
¼ cup tomato sauce
2 tsp capers
½ maple syrup or honey
Minced garlic
Minced ginger
2 Tbsp fresh grated
 coconut

Poultry

8 oz chicken
6 oz deli turkey

Seafood

4 oz salmon
4 oz skinless wild halibut
4 oz shrimp
4 oz scallops

Meats

4 oz bison sirloin steak
4 oz pork tenderloin

Vegetarian

4 oz tofu

Herbs & Spices

Parsley
Basil
Cinnamon
Nutmeg
Ground cloves
Ground red pepper
Dried oregano
Chili pepper flakes
Black pepper

Condiments

4 tsp honey
Balsamic vinegar
Rice wine vinegar
Dijon mustard

Making Good Food Choices

Use this template to guide you with your food choices
whether at home, at work, or out for dinner!

| Food Timing/HQ | Proportions | Portions | Nutrient Density |

Be strict with
starch portion.

If you are still hungry,
go for more vegetables
and then more protein.

Be strict with
fat portion.

Sample Day*

Meal	Starch	Fruit	Vegetables	Milk/ Yogurt/Soy	Lean Protein	Fat
Breakfast Coffee with skim milk	½ cup cooked steel cut oats with cinnamon			1 cup almond milk		7 choped walnuts
Snack			Celery with black pepper			8 cashews
Lunch Dress salad with balsamic vinegar and lemon juice			Spinach salad with tomatoes, roasted peppers, artichokes, hearts of palm, and red onion		4 oz. grilled chicken bread with oregano	¼ avocado
Snack Green tea				1 cup fat-free plain Greek yogurt with cinnamon		2 tsp natural peanut butter
Dinner			Steamed brussel sprouts, mixed green salad		6 oz.roasted cod with garlic, rosemary thyme and lemon	1 Tbsp vinaigrette on salad

*Start your day with a glass of warm water with lemon and drink 8 cups through the day along with 2 cups of green tea.

You may be a
B, S, S, L, D person!

Aim for 2 veggies,
for example, salad
and broccoli.

Add herbs and spices
to every meal!

More Options to Personalize Your Plan

To make this plan your own, start with the basic building blocks in the lists below: starches, proteins, milk (or milk substitute), fats, fruits, and of course, lots of vegetables. Then swap in all of your favorite foods using the portions in the lists, starting on the opposite page. The following are lists of some of my favorite foods to make it supereasy to shop and stock your pantry with healthy, delicious options! Products can change daily so please visit my Web site www.nutritiouslife.com for even more options.

Build a breakfast that includes:
Starch or fruit
Milk or milk substitute
Fat or protein

Build a morning snack that includes:
Fat or protein
Veggie

Build a lunch that includes:
Veggie
Protein
Fat
Starch (if you aren't having starch at dinner)

Build an afternoon snack that includes:
Milk or milk substitute
Fat

Build a dinner that includes:
Protein
Veggie
Fat
Starch (if you didn't have starch at lunch)

Starches

CEREALS
GENERIC   ½ cup
Arrowhead Mills Organic Old Fashioned Oatmeal Hot Cereal   ⅓ cup
Barbara's Bakery Puffins Original   ¾ cup
Barbara's Bakery Ultima Organic High Fiber Cereal   ½ cup
Bob's Red Mill Steel-cut oats   ¼ cup cooked
Ezekiel 4:9 Sprouted Whole Grain Cereal Original   ¼ cup
McCann's Irish Oatbran Hot Cereal   ¼ cup
Nature's Path Organic Flax Plus   ¾ cup
Nature's Path Organic Optimum Slim   ½ cup
Nature's Path Organic SmartBran with Psyllium & Oatbran   ¾ cup
Nutritious Living Hi-Lo 100% Natural Cereal   ½ cup
Quaker Instant Oatmeal   1 packet
Quinoa   ⅓ cup cooked
Uncle Sam   ½ cup
Uncle Sam Instant Oatmeal   1 packet

WAFFLES
GENERIC   1 waffle
Nature's Path Organic Waffles   1
Van's All Natural Multigrain Belgian Waffles   1
Van's Natural Foods Lite Totally Natural Waffle   1
Van's Natural Foods Organics with Vitamin Boost   1

BREAD AND TORTILLAS
GENERIC   1 slice bread, ½ pita, ½ English muffin, ½ roll or bun, 1 small tortilla
Arnold 100% Whole Wheat Sandwich Thins   1 sandwich thin
Damascus Bakeries Flax Roll-Up   1 roll-up
French Meadow Bakery Hemp Bread   1 slice
French Meadow Bakery Men's Bread   1 slice
La Tortilla Factory Smart & Delicious Low-Carb High-Fiber Tortillas   1 tortilla
Oroweat Sandwich Thins   1
Matthew's All Natural Whole Wheat English Muffin   1 muffin
Shiloh Farms Sprouted 7 Grain Bread, Organic   1 slice
Whole Wheat Pita Bread   ½ pita
Vermont Bread Company Whole Wheat Bread   1 slice

CRACKERS
Finn Crisp Original   4
Doctor Kracker Klassic Seed Flatbread   3/1
GG Scandinavian Bran Crispbread   5
Kavli Hearty Thick Crispbread   2
Mary's Gone Crackers Organic Original   4
Ryvita Dark Rye Crispbread   2
Wasa Fiber Crispbread   2

CHIPS AND STUFF
GENERIC   1 oz
Bearitos Organic No Salt No Oil Microwave Popcorn   5 cups, popped
Mary's Gone Crackers Sticks & Twigs   10 pieces
Newman's Own Organics Pop's-Corn No-Salt 94% Fat Free   3½ cups, popped

GRAINS
GENERIC   ⅓ cup
Brown rice   ⅓ cup cooked
Kamut   ⅓ cup cooked
Millet (whole)   ⅓ cup cooked
Quinoa   ⅓ cup cooked
Arrowhead Mills Pearled Barley   ⅓ cup cooked
Barilla Plus Pasta   ½ cup cooked
Bob's Red Mill 100% Whole Grain Quick Cooking Bulgur Wheat   ⅓ cup cooked
DeBoles Organic Whole Wheat Penne   ⅓ cup cooked
Eden Organic Soba Pasta   ½ cup cooked
Hodgson Mill Certified Organic Whole Wheat Fettuccine with Milled Flaxseed   ½ cup cooked
Ian's Panko Breadcrumbs, Whole Wheat   ¼ cup
Kretschmer Original Toasted Wheat Germ   3 Tbsp
Near East Long Grain & Wild Rice   ⅓ cup cooked
Near East Whole Grain Blends Brown Rice Pilaf   ⅓ cup cooked

STARCHY VEGETABLES
GENERIC ½–1 cup

Acorn squash ½ cup cooked

Butternut squash 1 cup cooked

Corn (ear) 1 small

Peas ½ cup

Potato (baked with skin) 1 small

Spaghetti squash 1 cup cooked

Sweet potato (baked with skin) 1 small

Amy's Organic Light in Sodium Split Pea Soup 1 cup

Dr. Praeger's Pancakes (Spinach, Broccoli, Sweet Potato) 1 pancake

Pacific Organic Light Sodium Creamy Butternut Squash Soup 1 cup

Imagine Organic Creamy Butternut Squash or Creamy Sweet Pea Soup 1 cup

LEGUMES
GENERIC ½ cup

Black beans ½ cup

Black-eyed peas ½ cup

Chickpeas ½ cup

Kidney beans ½ cup

Lentils ½ cup

Pinto beans ½ cup

Split peas ½ cup

White (cannellini) beans ½ cup

Amy's Organic Chili Medium Black Bean 1 cup

Tribe All Natural Hummus Classic 2 Tbsp

Milk or Milk Substitute

GENERIC 6 to 8 oz

Almond Dream (original) 8 oz

Dannon Oikos Greek Nonfat Yogurt 8 oz

Emmi Swiss Premium Lowfat Plain Yogurt 5.3 oz

Fage Total 0% Greek Yogurt (plain) 6 oz

Friendship Lowfat 1% Cottage Cheese ½ cup

Horizon Organic 1% Chocolate Milk 1 cup

Horizon Organic Skim Milk 1 oz

Lactaid Fat free Milk 1 cup

Light'n Lively lowfat Cottage Cheese ½ cup

Rice Dream Rice Drink 4 oz

Part-Skim Ricotta Cheese 3 oz

Silk Live! Soy Yogurt 8 oz

Silk Original Soymilk 8 oz

Soy DHA Omega-3 Milk 8 oz

Skim Plus Milk 1 cup

Stonyfield Oikos Plain Organic Greek Yogurt 8 oz

Stonyfield Organic Fat Free/Low-Fat Milk 4 oz

Tempt Original Hemp Milk 8 oz

WestSoy Lite Plain Soymilk Drink 8 oz

Vegetables

GENERIC No portion when there is no added fat

Alfalfa sprouts
Artichokes
Artichoke hearts
Arugula
Asparagus
Bamboo shoots
Bean sprouts
Beets
Broccoli
Brussels sprouts
Cabbage
Carrots
Cauliflower
Celery
Cherry tomatoes
Cucumber
Dandelion greens
Eggplant
Escarole
Green beans
Green onions/scallions

Hearts of palm
Iceberg lettuce
Jicama
Kale
Leeks
Mushrooms
Onion
Peppers, bell (green and red)
Radish
Romaine lettuce
Snow peas
Spaghetti squash
Spinach (cooked and raw)
Swiss chard
Tomato
Turnips
Water chestnut
Watercress
Yellow squash
Zucchini

Amy's Organic Chunky Vegetable Soup   1 cup
Bird's Eye Artichoke Hearts (frozen)   1 cup
Colavita Marinara Sauce   ½ cup
Healthy Delites Souffle (Roasted Vegetable, Zucchini, Spinach, or Broccoli)   1 souffle
Imagine Organic Light in Sodium Creamy Garden Broccoli Soup or Tomato Soup   1 cup
Imagine Natural Creamy Portobello Mushroom Soup   1 cup
Pacific Organic Light Sodium Creamy Tomato or Roasted Red Pepper and Tomato Soup   1 cup
Seapoint Farms Veggie Blends with Edamame   1 cup
V8 Juice   8 oz

FRUITS

GENERIC 1 small fruit or 1 cup cubes or berries

Apple   1 small
Apricot (dried)   9 halves
Apricot (fresh)   3 small
Banana   1 small
Blackberries   1 cup
Blueberries   1 cup
Cantaloupe   1 cup
Cherries   ½ cup
Figs   2 medium

Grapefruit   ½ fruit
Grapes (seedless)   15
Honeydew   1 cup
Kiwi   1
Mango   ½ medium
Mixed fruit cup   1 cup
Orange   1 medium
Papaya   1 cup
Passion fruit   3 medium
Peach   1 medium
Pear   1 small

Pineapple   1 cup
Plum   1 large
Pomegranate   ½ medium
Prunes   3
Raisins   ¼ cup
Raspberries   1 cup
Strawberries (sliced)   1 cup
Watermelon   1 cup
Santa Cruz Organic Apple Sauce   4 oz

Protein

POULTRY (3 to 4 oz)

Chicken breast

Cornish hen

Turkey breast

Aidells Chicken & Turkey Meatballs

Applegate Organics Roasted Chicken Breast (deli slices)

Applegate Organics Roasted Turkey Breast (deli slices)

Applegate Organics Turkey Bacon

Applegate Organics Turkey Burgers (frozen)

Bell & Evans Grilled Chicken Breasts (fully cooked, plain)

FreeBird Seasoned Grilled Chicken Breast Strips

Shady Brook Farms 93/7 Lean Ground Turkey

SnackMasters Range Grown Turkey Jerky, Original

FISH (3 to 4 oz)

Clams

Cod

Flounder

Halibut

Imitation crab (Surimi)

King crab

Lobster

Mahi mahi

Mussels

Red snapper

Salmon (wild)

Scallops (large sea)

Shrimp (fresh or frozen)

Sole

Swordfish

Trout

Tuna (bluefin, raw)

Tuna (canned chunk light in water), Tongol, Crown Prince

Tuna (fresh, cooked)

Henry & Lisa's Uncooked Natural Shrimp, Farm Raised

Sardines in Pure Spring Water

SnackMasters Natural Ahi Tuna Jerky

SnackMasters Natural Salmon Jerky

Whole Foods Whole Catch Wild Alaskan Sockeye Salmon Fillets (frozen)

St. Dalfour Ready to Eat Gourmet to Go Wild Salmon with Vegetables

MEAT (3 to 4 oz)

Beef, 95% lean ground

Beef, sirloin

Beef, T-bone

Beef, tenderloin

Canadian bacon

Ham, extra lean

Lamb loin

Pork, center loin chops

Pork, cutlet

Pork, tenderloin

Veal, loin

All Natural Great Range Brand Bison Patties

Applegate Organics Roast Beef (deli slices)

Laura's 92% Lean Frozen Ground Beef Patties

EGGS (2 eggs or 4 to 6 egg whites)

Eggology 100% Egg Whites

Eggology On-the-Go 100% Egg Whites

Country Hen Organic Omega-3 eggs

HOT DOGS AND SAUSAGES

Aidells Chicken & Apple Sausage

Applegate The Great Organic Uncured Chicken Hot Dog

Applegate The Great Organic Uncured Turkey Hot Dog

Applegate Organics Chicken and Apple Sausage

Bilinski's Organic or All Natural Chicken Sausage

Casual Gourmet Chicken Sausage

The Original Brat Hans Organic Breakfast Links Chicken Sausage

Wellshire Farms Chicken Sausage or Turkey Kielbasa

SOY OR MEATLESS PRODUCTS (3 to 4 oz)

Amy's California Veggie Burger

House Foods Tofu Steak Grilled

Lightlife Organic Tempeh

Woodstock Farms Organic Firm Tofu

Whole Foods Market Whole Kitchen Vegan Meatballs

LEGUMES

Black beans	½ cup
Black-eyed peas	½ cup
Chickpeas	½ cup
Kidney beans	½ cup
Lentils	½ cup

Pinto beans	½ cup
Split peas	½ cup
White (cannellini) beans	½ cup
Tribe All Natural Hummus	4 Tbsp

CHEESE

Cottage cheese (low-fat or fat-free)	½ cup
Feta cheese	3 oz
Goat cheese	3 oz
Mozzarella cheese	3 oz

Fats

OILS AND DRESSINGS

Coconut oil, Spectrum or Nutiva	2 tsp
Flaxseed oil	2 tsp
Grapeseed oil	2 tsp
Olive oil	2 tsp
Safflower oil	2 tsp
Salad dressing (oil-based)	1 Tbsp
Sesame seed oil	2 tsp
Sunflower oil	2 tsp
Walnut oil	2 tsp

OLIVES AND CHEESE

American cheese	1 slice (Note: higher in fat)
Goat cheese	1 oz
Olives (large)	6
Olives (small)	10
Parmesan cheese (grated)	3 Tbsp
Athenos Crumbled Feta	¼ cup
Athenos Reduced-Fat Crumbled Feta	¼ cup
Cabot 50% Reduced Fat Sharp Cheddar Cheese	1 oz
Cabot Reduced Fat with Omega 3 DHA	1 oz
Friendship All Natural Farmer Cheese	2 Tbsp
Horizon Organic Shredded Part-Skim Mozzarella Cheese	¼ cup
Horizon Organic Mozzarella String Cheese	1 stick
Organic Valley Stringles Part Skim Mozzarella Cheese	1
Mozzarella cheese	1 oz

NUTS, NUT BUTTERS, AND SEEDS

Almonds	8
Barney butter	2 tsp
Brazil nuts	2
Ground flaxseed	2 Tbsp
Hazelnuts	8
Nuttzo Nut Butter	2 tsp
Peanuts	15
Pecan halves	8
Pine nuts	1 Tbsp
Pistachio nuts	18
Pumpkin seeds	1 Tbsp
Sunflower seeds	1 Tbsp
Soy nuts	1 Tbsp
Walnut halves	7 or 1 Tbsp chopped
Arrowhead Mills Organic Valencia Peanut Butter	2 tsp
Blue Diamond Whole Natural Almonds 100 Calories Per Bag	1 pack
Carrington Farms Flax Paks	1 packet
Health Warrior Chia Seeds	2 Tbsp
Justin's All-Natural Classic Almond Butter	2 tsp
Justin's Organic Classic Peanut Butter	2 tsp
MaraNatha Organic Almond Butter	2 tsp
Naturally More Natural Peanut Butter	2 tsp
Smucker's Natural Peanut Butter	2 tsp

EGGS

Country Hen Organic Omega-3 Eggs	1 extra large
Horizon Organic Eggs	1
Land O Lakes Omega 3 All-Natural Eggs	1 large

FRUIT

Avocado	¼ medium

Acknowledgments

The New You and Improved Diet has been a decade in the making (or perhaps a lifetime!). A decade ago, I opened my nutrition practice and during that time, I have worked with and helped thousands of clients (who have also taught me a great deal) and created many lifelong friendships along the way. I am forever grateful to so many people, but I only have a couple pages so here goes...

Thank you to Maria Rodale and everyone at Rodale who tirelessly put their energy and efforts into making millions of lives better and healthier each day.

Thanks to Dave Zinczenko for the opportunity, again, to bring my passion to life. And to Steve Perrine, for making this book happen and for your continued support. A ginormous thank-you to my editor extraordinaire, Ursula Cary. I love working with you! Thank you to George Karabotsos whose brilliant design direction always makes things beautiful. To Nancy Bailey, Chris Rhoads, Mark Michaelson, Beth Lamb, Debbie McHugh, Yelena Nesbit, and the rest of the team at Rodale Books, thanks for ALL that you do!

A huge thank-you to *Women's Health*. I am honored to be part of such an extraordinary team. Michele Promaulayko, you inspire millions (including me) daily. Thank you for your friendship and for helping guide so many people to a place of better health. You rock!

I am lucky to have a team of people in my office that are truly like a second family. To all of you, thank you for your passion, commitment, energy, and enthusiasm for the ever-evolving field of nutrition as well as for your friendships. Karen Rogers, Lara Metz, Stacia Helfand, Amanda Buthmann, Tiffany Mendell, and Michelle Nabatian Routhenstein, one gigantic thank-you for the support, love, and dedication you bring on a daily basis. Thank you also to the interns who worked long and hard on this project: Hillary Appel, May Carr, and Leah Silberman.

Allison Keane, thank you for always believing in me, looking out for me, for your friendship and of course, for ALL of your hard work.

Sarah Mahoney, you are the writing ying to my yang! You continue to be the world's best writing partner. One day, we'll get to do all of this from an island! Therese Baran, thank you for being a superb creative, health junkie and creating recipes that we all want to eat!

Thank you to everyone at WME! Many thanks, once again, to Mel Berger, my literary agent. Can I still call you even if I am not writing a book? Thank you to Strand Conover and Jeff Googel for all of your very hard work, and also to Chris Dunn. Ken Slotnick, thank you for being the hardest-working and most supportive agent in the universe, and more important, thank you for making me smile every day.

It would not be possible to write this book without the support, guidance, and love of so many people including my incredible friends from all areas of my life to the many, many colleagues I am lucky enough to work with. Thank you. I hope you know who you are and I hope I thank you often enough. Hugs, kisses, and thanks to all of you.

Thank you Val Vaughan for being part of our family for so many years and loving my children with all your heart. Many thanks always to Brett Glassman. Thank you to my brother and sister in law, Judd and Samantha, for all that you have done over all of the years. Love you both.

Thank you Mom and Dad for continuing to parent just as intensely, passionately, and with as much love as when I couldn't even write my name let alone a book. I love you.

Rex and Maizy, you are the gifts that keep on giving. I don't know how it is possible but I love you more and more each day and one day you will understand that you teach me way more than I could ever possibly teach you. I love you more than the world.

Index

Underscored references indicate boxed text.